Trickling stream gurgles
brings music
    ... to dreams by night
dreams of days long past

Donations

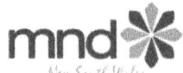

To support our vital work you can:
- visit us online at www.mndnsw.asn.au; or;
- call us on +61 2 8877 0999 Business Hours AEST

Motor Neurone Disease Association of New South Wales Inc
Australia, ABN 12 387 503 221

A Quality Life

The Memoirs of

June Burdon

(née Dollman)

15th June 1926 – 30th December 2003

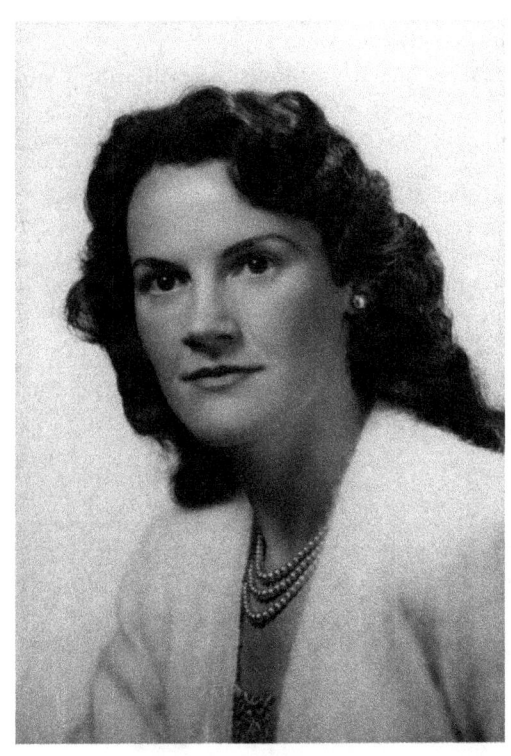

Copyright © 2003 June Burdon
Published: 2013, Trevor Burdon
Web: www.theburdons.com

Distribution
The paperback, ISBN 9780646904740, is printed on demand on orders from bookshops and online sellers. The ebook, ISBN 9781618429247, is available from online sellers only.

All rights reserved. Apart from any fair dealing for the purposes of private study, research, criticism, or review, as permitted under the Copyright Act, no part may be reproduced by any process without written permission. Enquiries should be addressed to the publishers.

National Library of Australia Cataloguing-in-Publication entry:
Author: Burdon, June, author.
Title: A quality life : the memoirs of June Burdon (nee Dollman)
15th June 1926 - 30th December 2003 /
June Burdon ; editor, Trevor Burdon ; illustrator, Peter Bublyk.
ISBN: 9780646904740 (paperback)
Notes: Includes index.
Subjects: Burdon, June
Amyotrophic lateral sclerosis — Patients — Biography.
Motor neurons — Diseases--Patients — Biography.
Neuromuscular diseases — Patients — Biography.
Other Authors/Contributors:
Burdon, Trevor, editor.
Bublyk, Peter, illustrator.
Dewey No: 616.8390092

Preface

The writing of *A Quality Life* gave June much pleasure, and in turn, it is remembered by her family as a great gift to them. In the making it gave context to her experiences, and we enjoyed sharing her recollections and uncovering the inevitable trivia that was brought to light. It is truly remarkable that she was able to recall so much of people and places and events. She always did know a lot about 'you' and that made for great conversation.

With the same keenness that she pursued all her activities, she worked under increasingly trying conditions to finish *A Quality Life*. She feared she wouldn't get there, but in her last moments rested contentedly. She had confirmed for herself, that to the last page she had said what she meant to.

It was discussed whether her biography be left verbatim, however I have respected June's preference for perfection. Early on she had agonised over style, though ultimately capturing the text a letter at a time took precedence. Hopefully it now conforms to a contemporary style, that is readable in both printed and ebook formats.

I thank my family, who helped with much transcription and collecting the photographs, ephemera and illustrations. Errol, especially, is to be thanked for his tireless care, and moreover for reaching out 'to touch her shoulder during the nights when I became aware that she was awake - a small gesture hopefully reassuring her that although she was isolated, she was not alone.'

Inspired by June, I turned my mind to a late night haiku. I encourage you to try it yourself sometime. In honour of a wonderful mother:

> *Thunder crackles loud*
> *precipitating soft rain*
> *creek gurgles birds coo*

Trevor Burdon, 19th December 2011.

Family tree

Charles John Dollman
b. 1817 Islington, Middlesex, England
m. 1842 Islington, England
d. 1860 Adelaide, SA

Eliza Harriett Parmeter
b. 1822
d. 1876 John St Hospital, North Adelaide, SA

Charles Alexander Dollman
b. 1844 Islington, Middlesex, England
d. 1888 England

William Parmeter Dollman
b. 1845 St George's, Hanover Sq
d. 1908 Adelaide, SA

Walter Dollman
b. 1847 Clapham, Surrey
d. 1916 Adelaide, SA

Edith Dollman
b. 1850 Working, Surrey
d. 1937 Wangaratta, Vic

Henry Herbert Dollman
b. 1852 Working, Surrey
d. 1934

Ruth Dollman
b. 1854 Currie St, Adelaide, SA
m. 1877
d. 1919

Ernest Guy Dollman
b. 1857 137 Hindley St, Adelaide, SA
m. 1885 St Lukes, Adelaide, SA
d. 1931 Unley, Adelaide, SA

Francis Guy Dollman
b. 1858 74 Hindley St, Adelaide, SA
m. 1885
d. 1933

Doris Dollman
b. 1888 Wilcannia, NSW
m. 1914 Wilcannia, NSW
d. 1957

Ruth Dollman
b. 1890 Wilcannia, NSW
d. 1894

Guy Herbert Dollman
b. 1892 Goonalga Station, Wilcannia, NSW
m. 1920 St Lukes, Adelaide, SA
d. 1967 Adelaide, SA

Robert Rogers
b. Unknown Unknown
d. Unknown Unknown

Jane Rogers
b. 1855 Ireland
d. 1929 Adelaide, SA

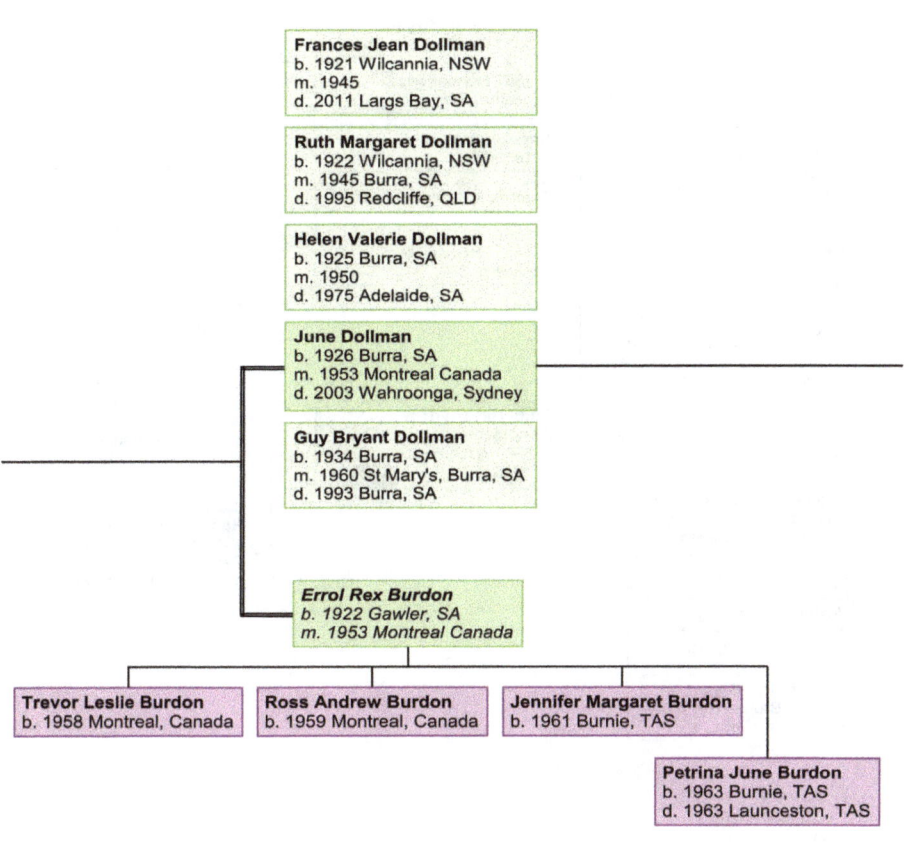

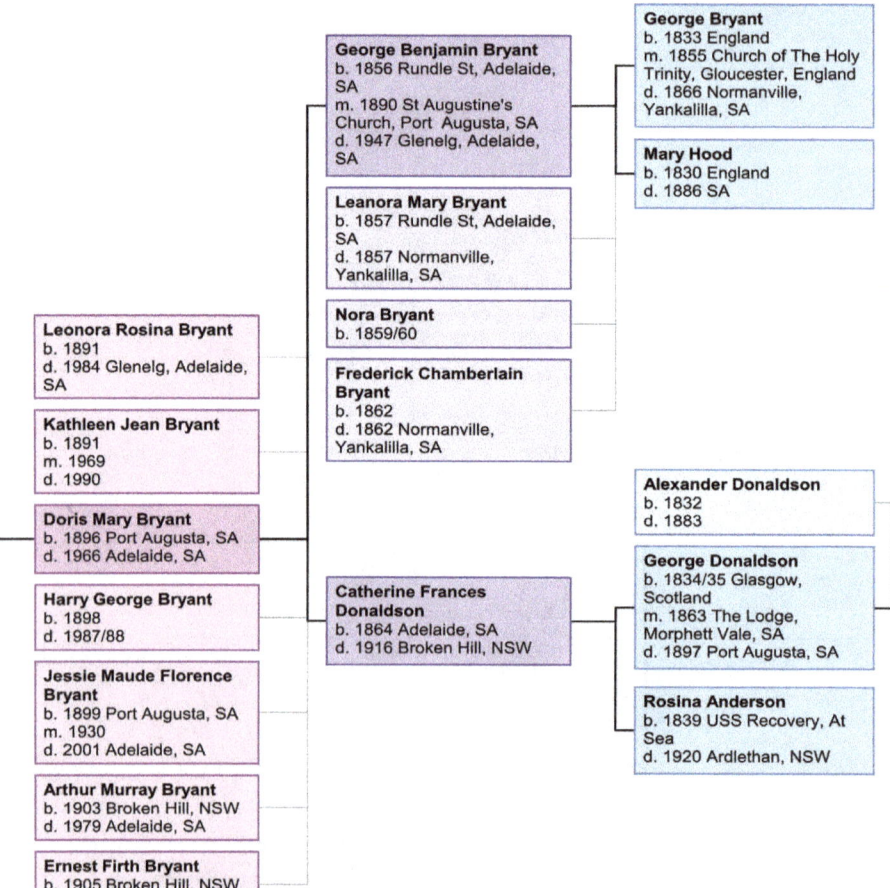

iv

Timeline of events

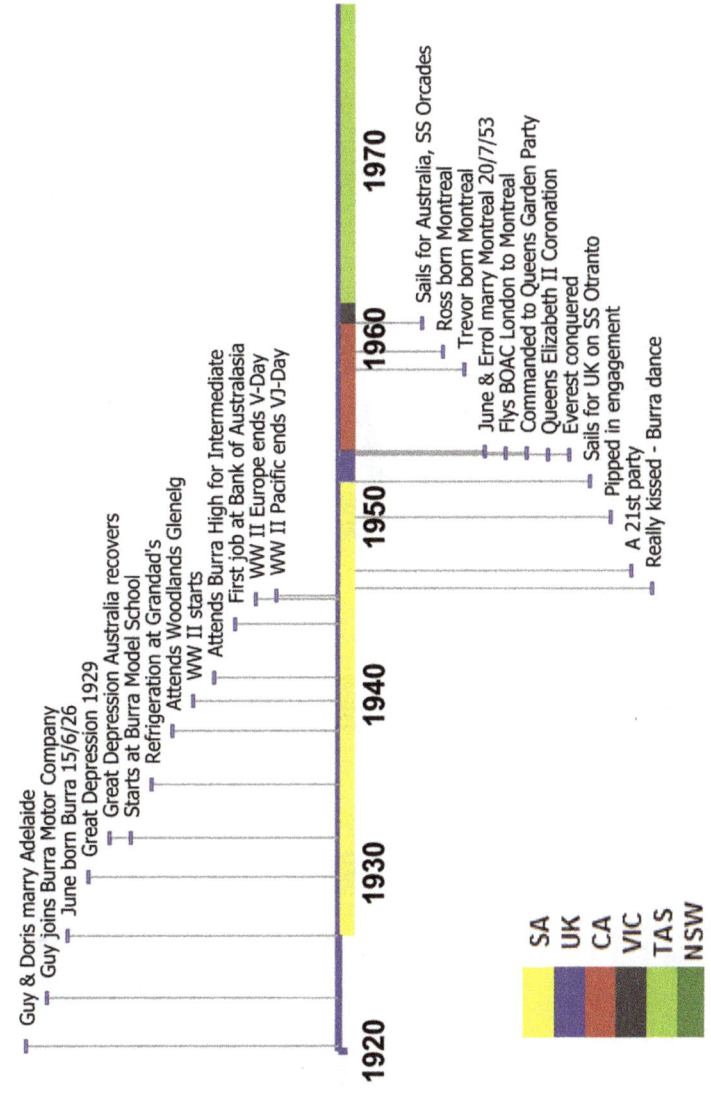

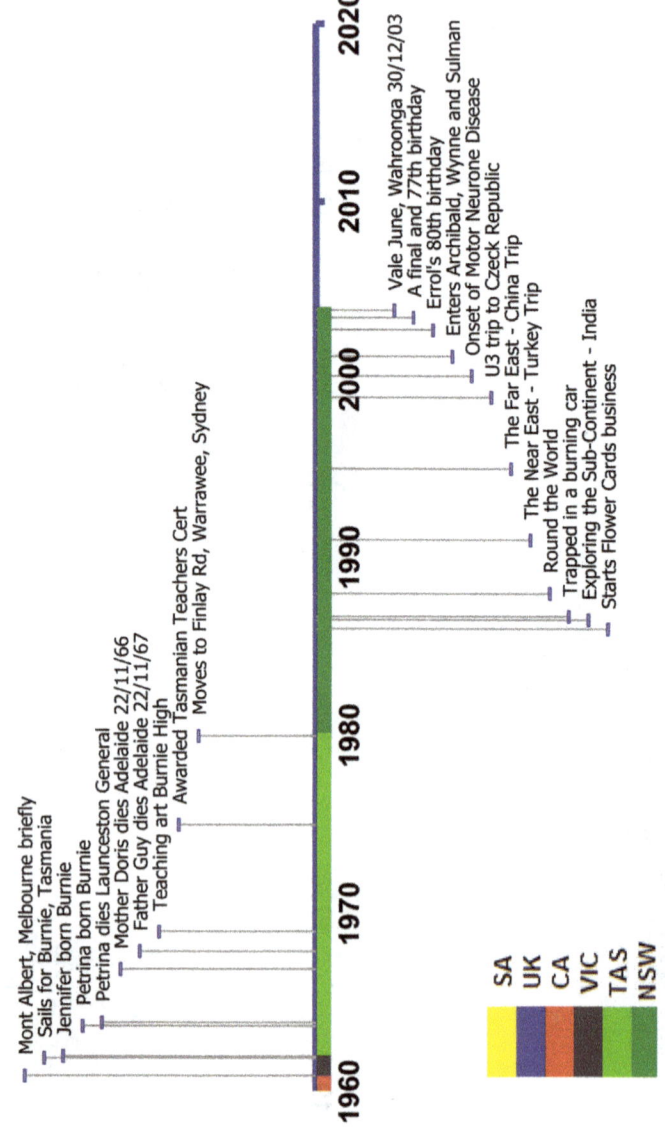

Contents

Preface i
    Family tree ii, Timeline of events v

The Month of June 1

Early Recollections 3
    St Mary's – the social centre of town 4, Favourite games 6

Doris and Guy Dollman, Burra 9
    The Burra Motor Company 9, Dad's interests 11, The Burra Burra Mine & District 12, Ware Street, Kooringa 12, 6 Queen Street, Kooringa 14

Childhood and Teens 17
    Chop picnics and singalongs 18, Family shopping 18, My closest friend 20, Christmas, birthdays & holidays 20, Holidays in Adelaide 21, Simple delights 22, 8 Broadway, Glenelg 23, The Ice-Man cometh 24, The secret Renault 24, A chauffeur at our disposal 25, Summer holidays 25

Schooling 29
    Burra Model School 29, Woodlands CEGGS 32, Burra High School 39

The War Years 41
    Our war effort 41, Boys, boys, boys! 44, I join the workforce 46, Weekends in Adelaide 47, My sisters marry 48, V-Day – the end of the War 49

After the War 51
    Dances, dresses and courtship 52, To venture abroad 69, Life on the high seas 72

Photo Pages I 80

The United Kingdom! 93
    Arrival in London 93, York Gate 94, Jobs for Rae and Me 95, Backpacking 96, Living at the Strand Palace Hotel 100, Getting to know England 103, Art at St Martin's 107, The Beaufort Hunt 108, Visiting Jess and Skipper at St Albans 110, Girlfriends 113, Plans to marry 115, The Coronation of Queen Elizabeth 116, Preparing for married life 117, A Royal Garden Party 119, I missed my flight! 121

Canada - Reunited with Errol 125
A Montreal wedding 126, Honeymoon at Château Laurier 127, Our first home together 132, Settling in to Montreal 135, A most lovely apartment - Monkland Avenue 145, Starting a family 155, Son No. 2 159

Photo Pages II 162

Return to Australia 175
The voyage home 175, Melbourne and pregnant again 178

Tasmania 181
25 Seaview Avenue 184, Jennifer joins us 188, Petrina June ... briefly 193, Settled for eighteen years 197, My teaching career 203, Our children grow up 208, Returning to study 210, Friends in Tasmania 212, Rita Simpson 212, Transfer to Parklands 213, Holidays from Tasmania 214, Errol leaves Tioxide 216

Sydney, New South Wales 219
Baldwin St International 222, More language studies 226, My locked knee 227, Trapped in a burning car 227, Flower Cards of Australia 229, Holidays from Sydney 230, Flinders Island 232, Round the world - Egypt, Europe and North America 235, Exploring the sub-continent – our India trip 238, The Near East – our Turkey trip 241, The Far East – our China trip 244, Other travels 253

My Silent Years 255
The Onset of MND 255; Against all odds - entering the Wynne 261, Eighty-six thousand words 262, Haikus from nature 262, The Old Bugger's Eighty 265, My 77th birthday party 266

Index 269

The Month of June

Dusk was falling fast and the days were getting shorter in the chilly winter of 1926. It was the 15th June in the small town of Burra Burra, 100 miles north of Adelaide in South Australia. Frances, then aged five, recalls Auntie Kath phoning Guy to hurry home in order to light the kerosene lights, as Doris was about to give birth to her fourth child. Then followed a call to Dr David Steele, who was the family doctor - one of two resident in the town. Later that evening Dr Steele delivered a baby girl, the fourth daughter for Guy and Doris Dollman. As she had done for all previous births, Kathleen Bryant, Doris' elder sister and a trained nurse, travelled from Adelaide to assist in the delivery.

For the fourth time the parents hoped for a boy, and so the latest arrival remained unnamed for some time. They were at a loss for a name until they decided on the obvious, June - the month of birth and a popular name that year.

Having no second name like her sisters was a source of considerable frustration throughout June's childhood. Especially when, aged twelve, June entered a new school and on being asked her name had to admit to having no second name - 'Just plain June.' Her new classmates could not believe such misfortune, and she felt as though it was considered as severe a handicap as having only one leg. More particularly as they were all blessed with exotic names like Nadine, Nanette, Maxine, Nina, Annette, Poppy, Sylvia, Deidre and Cynthia as well as equally exciting second names.

To make matters worse, her sisters avoided such humiliation as they were christened with more desirable names. Frances Jean, called 'Fuff' by Peg who as a child could not pronounce Frances, and so remained Fuff to family and friends from then on. Ruth Margaret whose cousin was also christened Ruth became 'Peg', a common diminutive for Margaret, became known as Peg all of her life. Her immediately older sister, born a year earlier, was christened Helen Valerie.

Early Recollections

Despite my handicap, it was a happy childhood - unlike many others in the town. Doris and Guy were devoted and loving parents, who did not spoil their children but bestowed many advantages other families could not afford. It was during the Depression, but strangely, as we grew older we girls could not remember anything of consequence about it. As we remembered all children had shoes, though often they were shabby and sometimes had holes in the soles. Certainly there were the swaggies, who wandered from town to town with their swags, rolled blankets with tied jangling mugs and plates. They went from door to door asking for work - chopping firewood was common - and were recompensed with a few coins, and usually a cup of tea and something to eat. They were polite and usually welcomed as they were never a threat to housewives or children. Frances, however, remembers one occasion when Mum gave a sandwich to a man who threw it away as soon as he got out of sight. No doubt he was expecting money, not food for which he had asked.

The Dollman family never did without the essentials; we had good wholesome food and were always very well dressed. Mum would sit night after night, often till two in the morning, sewing by kerosene lamp with her hand operated Wertheim sewing machine. She turned out beautiful clothes for her four daughters, often in pairs, two matching for the older girls, and two matching for the younger girls. Mum had no training in sewing but with patterns was very adept at making dresses, hats and bloomers. All were made in matching materials, which were often supplied by Auntie Kath and billed to Grandfather Bryant!

Fuff has recounted some details of my birth, as she was then five years old. My earliest memory must have been when I was three years old, as Dad's mother, Jane (Grandma Dollman) died in September 1929. She was lying in my parents' bed, not long before her death, and Fuff says she gave me a huge one-pound block of Cadburys chocolate, wrapped in the recognisable purple and gold paper - indeed very regal and much prized by a child. I also have vivid memories of a small doll dressed in lavender, but it would be unlikely that I received two such presents at this time.

Grandma and Grandad moved from Wilcannia, and were staying with us for a time before going on to live in Adelaide with their only living daughter Doris. She was older than Dad by four years, and a sister Ruth born between the two had died aged five from a tooth infection caused by an abscess. Surprisingly, Dad and his sister did not get on, as she was very bossy and being the older felt superior. Doris thrust her opinions and advice on my mother and insisted on passing-on her used pram and baby things, depriving Mum the pleasure of choosing her own for the newly born, which Mum rather resented, Dad and Jack Glennister, however were good friends.

St Mary's – the social centre of town

As in most country towns, the church at Burra was the main centre for social gatherings. Concerts and community functions were generally held in the local Institute, which also served as the picture theatre on Saturday night. There was no shortage of entertainment and many chances to wear pretty clothes, which were much admired by all the townspeople. All the Dollmans attended St Mary's Church of England each Sunday, and we children went to Sunday School until our teens.

From 1933-1939, St Mary's Minister was Donald Redding. Being rather rotund, he was lovingly called 'Pop', which he encouraged with the children of the parish. He was popular among the adults and on his ministerial rounds loved to lick the spoon if there was a cake in the making, a passion the ladies happily indulged him in. Possibly in his early thirties, he was a bachelor and remained so all his life. (Mum told me years later that she believed he had a fondness for Mrs Dow.) Living in the vicarage with him were two young men, Jack Pengilley who moved from Kangaroo Island, and Clem Davey, a local music teacher. Clem became the church organist after Graham Dow left the town. Years later, Peg and my friend Rae learnt piano from him and both admitted to falling for him. Pop Redding was liked by all in the community, for he joined the men in the pubs where he drank lemonade and took the local boys swimming in the mine pool. At least one of those groups included my future husband, who, when about twelve, remembers Pop supervising a group of them of all denominations.

The local boys used to climb down the old, dangerous and uncovered mine shafts. I clearly recall the time a Methodist minister fell to his death, when attempting to cover a shaft to prevent the boys going down to collect bird eggs. My future husband was one of the boys, who participated in this perilous pastime. He later told me of the exploits of the local daredevil, Jimmy James, who constantly put his life at risk by climbing further down the shafts than anyone else, and with legs dangling like a foolhardy frog, then dived into the pools of unknown depth below.

In 1939 at the start of the war, Donald Redding joined up as a Major and gained a reputation as an 'orright ozzy guy', and was well known throughout the forces. After the war, he returned to the ministry as the Bishop of Willochra, and visited Burra for confirmations. Graham Dow was organist during and after Pop's term. Always a jokester, while the congregation filed in and between playing hymns, he used to slip in nursery rhymes like Mary had a Little Lamb, Little Jack Horner and so on.

After Sunday School we children walked home together. In the season when the grapes were ripening on our neighbour's vines and ready for harvest, a favourite pastime was to go through the hole in the fence and have a luscious feed. This was much more exciting than asking and a challenge not to be observed by the owners. So much for our Christian upbringing!

One day Diana Dow was not well and went home ahead of us. When we arrived home, there was no Diana so our worried parents set up a search. Eventually Diana turned up unhurt. She had been enticed under a bridge by an 'odd' man, and neighbour, who had simply 'touched' her. We were all warned to be careful, but nothing more was done as he was regarded as being just a bit retarded and harmless. Now I am dubious, as I recall when playing in our back yard and aged about four, the same man had called me to the back dividing fence and asked me to go behind a shed and to pull my pants down. Although he was on the other side of the fence, I was suspicious, refused to do so and ran away. Paedophilia was not thought of and unheard of in our early lives - or so I believe. We were simply told not to go off with strange men.

Favourite games

In those days we enjoyed simple games involving no cost, but we were inventive and so happy. When three or four years old I loved making mud pies as children did in those days. It's surprising as I was always very fussy and Mummy was so particular about clean clothes ... but expect I was well set up with dirt, water, pie dish and a pinny.

As younger children we all inherited Fuff's dolls pram and other toys, but not her beautiful celluloid doll, which she still has sitting on her bed in her 80th year. Just as well we did not have it to play with!

I remember drawing a large house plan with all the rooms and passages with a stick on the ground. Most backyards were dirt in Burra, and lawns were rare. Then with a friend, we'd play house by going from room to room with our dolls, sweeping with toy brooms, and setting tea parties with the kindergarten table and chairs, which my very clever Daddy had made for Fuff and Peg.

We also played school, with me the teacher of course, and usually Diana Dow the pupil. From then on, I always wanted to be a teacher. I can still remember smacking her, as that must have been what I thought teachers did. I had yet to meet Miss Pearce but perhaps had heard about her. Although two months younger, Diana started school a year before me and was always a year ahead. My vivid memories are of the many times her brothers used to insist that Diana was the elder, which I knew was not so. They took great pleasure from teasing me.

EARLY RECOLLECTIONS

Playing 'Doctors and Nurses' with friends or dolls was all very harmless and not at all sexual. Hopscotch, skipping with rope, and marbles continued into our teens, though the latter was mainly a boy's game. We also used tin cans tied to our feet for stilts. When Guy came along, Daddy made toys such as wagons and building blocks for him. These were used later by the grandchildren when visiting.

It is interesting that my early ambition was to be a teacher, then architect, then writer and finally most of all lawyer - as I loved arguing, as my family will endorse. As there was no money for any of us to go to university, the latter was unachievable. Though not exactly a game, one could say I was playing florist when I picked the wildflowers that grew nearby on the hills, just up from Thames Street. At other times I picked from our garden, tied them up in little bouquets and sold them to the neighbours for thrippence (three pence). All profits went to a church charity - no doubt an overseas mission or hospital. I think this was in my pre-school years. At the same time, and in following years, I entered wildflower arrangements in the spring Burra Show. Not surprisingly, I have also had desires to be a florist, but have settled for gardening and painting flowers.

Doris and Guy Dollman, Burra

My mother, Doris Mary Bryant, was one of the seven children of Catherine Frances Donaldson, who died in 1916 when Doris was aged twenty. Catherine bore George Benjamin Bryant seven children: four daughters and three sons over a span of fourteen years from 1891-1905 - with one can imagine, a few miscarriages in between. Doris met my father, Guy Herbert Dollman, when she took up her first and only teaching position in Wilcannia, New South Wales. She had done her training in Sydney as at the time her family was living in Broken Hill. Though inside NSW, in those days it was unofficially regarded as part of South Australia as Adelaide was the closest capital city.

Doris and Guy were married in 1920 in Adelaide, where her father and family had since returned. When she was twenty-four and he twenty-eight, they started their married life in Wilcannia, and Guy assisted his father in the general store. Frances and Ruth were born there, and in 1924 they moved to Burra where Helen and I were born, making four girls within five years plus two miscarriages. Seven and a half years later, on 30th January 1934, a son Guy Bryant joined the family. This was indeed a happy event. Little Guy was cuddled and worshipped by his adoring sisters and became thoroughly spoiled. He was smothered with love.

The Burra Motor Company

In 1923 Dad joined his brother-in-law Jack Glennister in his motor business, The Burra Motor Company. The automobile business was growing fast in the mid-twenties and the company thrived under the partnership, selling new cars, gasoline, spare parts, and doing maintenance and repairs. Early in the fifties, it extended to selling some electrical goods. After only a few years, Jack Glennister, his wife Doris (Dad's sister), and two daughters Ruth Grace and Mary Elizabeth moved to Adelaide, and so the partnership ended. Dad carried on, ably assisted by Graham Dow in the office for possibly ten years. At the height of the business, fifteen men were employed by the company.

Over time, other businesses (at least eight) traded under the general name of garage, offering services related to the motor industry.

Dad and worked night and day, six or seven days a week, and took only one holiday in his late fifties. Although he provided well for his family, he never made a fortune, as he was too generous. He always felt sorry for the poor old farmers, whom he said were having bad times. He never pressed them for payment, and consequently, he often was not paid at all. Despite long working hours, he was always smiling, cheerful, and was loved and respected by his employees and all the district - not to mention his family. His three sisters-in-law Nora (Leonora), Kath and Jess simply adored him, and his three brothers-in-law Harry, Arthur and Firth treated and loved him like a brother.

Dad did make time, as most menfolk did in the country, to visit one of the local pubs around 5:30 p.m. before the 6:00 p.m. closing. For most of his life, it was The Commercial Hotel, which was then right next door to his first premises. In fact, when Fuff fulfilled her ambition to be Dad's office girl, she reported that there was a hole in the wall through which drinks were supplied to the workers and the boss while working late. These gatherings at the pub were really social occasions for men to discuss the affairs of the day, and for companionship. (The womenfolk had many opportunities with their afternoon teas and their church and school meetings and functions). In those early days, women were not allowed in the bar but had to go into the Ladies Lounge. Generally, a lady did not frequent such places unless travelling on a hot day, and then more often than not her husband would bring a cold drink to the car or other mode of transport. Part of his demanding work came at night or in the early hours of the morning, when he was constantly on call as the RAA (Royal Automobile Association) representative for after-hours breakdowns. These calls were numerous and Guy would have to get out of bed on chilly mornings to attend the unfortunates, who had trudged to the nearest town and pulled publicans out of bed in order to phone through. Thirty years on, one of his loyal and reliable mechanics, Jeff Neale, agreed to take over this thankless job and did it for thirty-five years.

Dad's interests

Somehow, Guy found time for his main interests. He was a passionate photographer, taking many photographs of his children, family and church picnics, scenes and special town occasions. He developed and enlarged his photographs in a dark room within his workroom. He was a very able self-taught wood craftsman. For their first children he made a cradle, high chair and a rocking horse. For their home, he made two console tables that were used as desks, (one cedar and one mahogany), a mahogany traymobile, and bedside or lounge tables as the need arose. Most cherished were two beautiful and intricately made lounge chairs - then known as Morris chairs. They had mahogany frames, wide arms, upholstered seats, and backs slatted behind for height adjustment. They were very comfortable, solid, and most attractive pieces of furniture that the family regrets selling during some refurbishment of the dining room. For some thirty years or more, they had sat either side of the fireplace as 'his and hers'.

Dad worked at night in his workroom at home, particularly in the early years of marriage when good furniture was much needed. More complicated work was done in the garage workshop, where he could avail himself of the tools and equipment.

Dad's principal talent and enjoyment was singing, having a rich baritone voice admired by all who had the privilege of hearing him. Throughout his life, he was soloist in St Mary's Church choir and was in great demand for all major functions in the surrounding districts, such as when the State Governor or other notable persons visited. When the singing teacher of Peter Dawson, the renowned baritone, heard him sing, he wanted to have Dad as his pupil. Dad was asked to compere concerts, and during World War II arranged parties in the district, raising funds for the war effort. He loved singing and was a natural compere, having a great sense of humour and personality. He loved opera and operettas, singing arias at home and work. To everyone's surprise, and even his own, he enjoyed Bing Crosby's crooning and began to sing the tunes Bing made popular like South of the Border - though not quite in Bing's style!

The Burra Burra Mine & District

When Dad, Mum, Fuff and Peg moved to Burra Burra, the town was a thriving pastoral and agricultural district with an interesting history. Copper had been discovered there and in 1845, the Burra Burra Mine opened. For years it was the world's richest copper mine and it was the first mineral mine in Australia. It was boom time for the State and copper mining saved it from bankruptcy. Six hundred teamsters were engaged to drive ten times as many bullocks, (and later mules), to haul copper to Port Wakefield for shipping to Europe. The mine was worked for the next 32 years, but production slowed as the water table was reached, and was then completely overshadowed by the discovery of gold in the eastern states. There was an exodus of the Cornish miners and Welsh smelters, who had originally rushed to work in the Burra mine. Gradually, the sheep, wool and wheat industries took over.

Burra Burra district, nestled in a basin surrounded by hills consisted of four hamlets, Aberdeen, Redruth, Hampton and Copperhouse, and the company town known as Kooringa. Later the district was abbreviated to Burra, and the hamlets Aberdeen and Redruth became Burra North, being about a mile north of Kooringa, with the mine between the two.

Ware Street, Kooringa

My parents and sisters first lived in Thames Street, Kooringa, in one of the original 'Company' cottages; it was here that Helen was born. I was born in Ware Street in a comfortable six-room house with a passage running from the front door to the back. On the left of the passage was our parents' bedroom. On the right was the sitting room that led into Fuff and Peg's bedroom. The passage ran into the dining room with a breakfast room to the left and a third bedroom for Helen and me off the dining room on the right. At the back there was a covered verandah on the left of which was the kitchen with a wood stove for most of the cooking. There was also kerosene stove in the breakfast room for lighter meals and making tea. Having no sink, washing up was done in a large bowl and emptied outside. At the other end of the verandah was the bathroom. A few steps led down to the yard with a laundry on the right. Here all dirty clothes were prepared for the weekly wash on Sunday night. The copper was filled with white items soaking in Reckitt's Blue and then set with wood, ready to be lit early Monday morning. All whites, handkerchiefs and cottons were boiled. We always had a washerwoman, and as well, Mummy always did a daily wash of our day-to-day underclothes and frocks. With four little girls there was a lot to be washed, and unlike today, we wore frocks that needed to be ironed. Especially as we wore fresh clothes with never a stain. We all remember the time, when all ready to set out on a holiday, eager little Helen rushed out with a forgotten tin of honey. She dropped it, resulting in honey going everywhere and all over her!

In the yard, we had a huge underground cellar for cool storage, and as we had no running water, the usual country rainwater tank supplied our household needs. Water was heated on the wood stove for washing and baths etc. My mother was very particular about bathing. When we were little, every night we washed in a big tin bath in front of the wood stove. Fuff can remember Dad coming home some nights in time to dry us. I also recall on cold nights, when we were not well, that we were bathed by the wood fire in our bedroom - we had fireplaces in most rooms. When we grew older, we bathed in a normal bath in the bathroom. As water was always scarce, we usually shared the water, but as I did not like that practice I was always spoilt and permitted to go first! On occasions of extreme water shortage, we solved that problem by standing in the bath with a large bowl of water on a plank across the bath, washing ourselves and then pouring the water over us.

As was normal in most country towns and many city homes too, there were no 'mod cons'. We had no water laid on and no electricity; lighting was by kerosene lamps and candles. Later we had a wonderful pressurised petrol lamp, which hung from the centre of sitting room ceiling and when lit made a terrifying 'whoosh' as though about to explode. It was our pride and joy, and each night Daddy stood on a chair to light it.

The lavatory was in the back yard and 'potties' were placed discreetly under our beds. They were used by those too scared to go outside and face the 'bogey-man' - though small children thought he could be hiding under the bed! Another terror for all ages was finding the deadly red-back spider, which loved to nest in the warm atmosphere underneath the lavatory seat. This particular spider bred prolifically and was very common in the hot, dry mid-north area of SA.

6 Queen Street, Kooringa

A year or so after Guy was born we moved to Queen Street, also in Kooringa, to a much larger house which we thought was a mansion. It had eight indoor rooms: four bedrooms, sitting and dining room, breakfast room, kitchen with pantry, bathroom with septic toilet (!); and Dad's outside workroom accessible from the back verandah. There was another small two-room building with the laundry and a small playroom. At the back door, there was a huge covered verandah where Guy slept when he was young, and where we all loved to sleep from time to time. Here Dad installed a basin where he shaved with hot water from the stove in the morning, and washed himself when he came home from work. Underneath the verandah was a door to an enormous cellar running under the kitchen and pantry. The entrance to the steps was enclosed with a picket fence where Mum had a raised display of pot plants and ferns. Apart from the one curious visit, we never visited the back cellar. I know that I for one did not venture very far as there were cobwebs everywhere down there. There was another cellar under the house from the front verandah. As children, we sometimes played there to escape the heat when shade temperatures rose well over the 100 °Fahrenheit (38.4 °C). On many occasions, it was as high as 117 °F (48°C). On one such occasion when Fuff was working for Dad, she recalls he would not let her go to the office so she spent two days reading Gone With The Wind, an epic of 1000 pages, by candlelight.

The pièce de résistance was the outside lavatory with two seats together and a separate lower one for a child - a three-holer - the envy of our friends! Our outdoor lavatories were always scrubbed out after the weekly wash, with the leftover boiling water from the copper. No water was ever wasted.

This house had been designed by an architect and built by a wealthy landowner in the district, Mr McBride. Originally, it had its own gas supply, the only one in the district, but it had been converted to electricity before our time. Rather elegant gas lamps still hung in the bedrooms and living rooms, and aroused much curiosity.

The previous tenant was widowed with several children, and took in male boarders - a customary source of income for a widow.

When Fuff was transferred to Renmark, she met and married Bob Breeze, who had a fruit block there. Mum sometimes visited her, and also had short holidays with Auntie Nora at Glenelg. Once I was the only girl cared for at home, Mum religiously cleaned and polished the house and stained the floor either side of the carpet down the long passage.

The house was set on a large block with spare land at the back where we kept 'chooks'. There was a very nice garden in front with a small rose garden and arch, agapanthus, golden rod, lilac and verbena trees. Mum loved gardening but it was a struggle to keep seedlings alive in the hot weather. Faced with a constant shortage of water, hand watering her garden was a slow and pleasant pastime on balmy summer evenings. We all tried to help with the weeding, planting and general maintenance. I recall weeding the front garden with the aid of my then boyfriend Frank Storey. I do not know if it was appreciated as my mother was very particular, as was I, and she was very hard to please. Despite this we all loved her dearly and she us.

Childhood and Teens

Our parents did much entertaining, including bridge parties and singalongs around the pianola. Most of our parents' friends were musically inclined and immediate neighbours or parishioners of St Mary's Church.

Fuff recalls the excitement when the magnificent upright pianola arrived brand-new from Adelaide and was hoisted up onto the front verandah of the house - though I was too young to remember the occasion. We were all fascinated by the technology, no doubt German, where the operator had only to press the foot pedals to make a music roll revolve and operate the linked keys. The music played while displaying the score and words on the rolls. The pianola looked exactly like a normal upright piano: same size, full keyboard, beautiful tone, and could be played by a non-pianist. From Adelaide, our many pianola rolls were stored together with our gramophone records in a beautiful cabinet carved by our clever father.

Mummy told us that when they first arrived in Burra, 'visiting cards' were in common usage. The ladies of the town would send notes to a new arrival, announcing that they wished to visit and make her acquaintance - providing that she was socially suitable! The newly arrived would then send her card, announcing the time and day when she would be 'at home'. In return, the visitors would leave their cards with their at-home information. A wonderful way to make new friends! (I do not know when this custom stopped, as I was never aware of it while I was growing up.)

Throughout my mother's life, she rarely addressed a woman friend by her Christian name - only as Mrs 'So-and-So'. The exceptions were ladies she had known since childhood. She caused quite a stir when she called the new Minister's wife 'Molly', as Molly's family had been close friends of the Bryants. We children, then in our teens, also did so as she was quite young. The men however, called each other by their Christian names.

Chop picnics and singalongs

Like our parents, much of our lives revolved around Church, Sunday School and picnics at the Gorge where we swam and played in the pool, and had memorable 'Chop Picnics'. The children gathered wood, eucalyptus twigs and leaves for the fire over which lamb chops and sausages were cooked by the men. Salads and cakes were prepared by the women. These were the forerunners of the barbecue. There is no smell quite like the smoky aroma of the bush, and of lamb cooked on a fire of eucalyptus leaves.

There were other picnics to Baldina Station owned by the Barker family. For such outings, those without cars travelled in Alec Bevan's bus or piled into the back of utilities and trucks supplied by the farmers. It was great fun, though somewhat hot and dusty, as most of the roads were just dirt.

On Sundays, we visited our friends the Pellews and Marchants on their nearby farms, and the Norman Pearces at the Gums station. In the evening were the singalongs with Mrs Hann at the piano and though Mummy played well she was outshone, and usually retired into the background while the former accompanied Dad for concerts.

All the Hann family were musical. Mrs Hann had a studio in her home where she taught dancing, music and other artistic pursuits. As I had an 'obvious talent' for dancing and showing-off, she offered to teach me all the way to stardom! I trudged up to her home on Hill Street overlooking the town, and though I enjoyed it, I did not go beyond tap-dancing the Highland Fling, Sailors' Hornpipe and other favourites.

Family shopping

The shops were open for trading on Friday evenings when it was time for family shopping, or for teenagers to just get out and meet friends. When we were younger, Mummy usually went alone rather than drag us all around. On these occasions while living in Ware Street, Miss Ward who lived behind us came to baby-sit; or Fuffy was put in charge. Fuffy was very caring and conscientious, and as the eldest child took her responsibilities seriously. Often too seriously, Helen and I thought, especially as we got older and tended to run a bit wild - doing things that we preferred our parents not to know! A heavy burden is placed on the eldest child.

All groceries, meat, bread and milk were delivered to the home. Each day we phoned the butcher and often the grocer, and shortly afterwards our orders would be delivered by the 'grocer boys', so called, regardless of age. For many years our grocer boy was Rex Opperman, a champion in South Australia and Victoria, and a nephew of the world-famous cyclist Hubert Opperman.

The baker's cart called daily with freshly baked bread, normally only white and brown, high top or flat, and lovely sweet smelling yeast buns. There was a regular 'baker's dozen' that was thirteen, and invariably children who hung around the cart were given a free bun. Hence the arrival of the baker's cart was greeted with great excitement.

The greengrocer likewise called with his cart, and the housewife made her choice. In addition, growers came around regularly selling fruit and vegetables. Each morning and evening, we hung a billycan on the gate, and our milkman doing his rounds filled it with the desired amount of fresh cow's milk. In those days milk was not pasteurised, so it was placed in a bowl on the wood stove and slowly brought to boil until the cream rose to the top. When cool a lovely crusty cream formed, which was delicious served with desserts, or with jam on scones or bread.

Bences, Drew & Crewes, and Matthews all stocked the latest in ladies and mens fashions, as well as materials, haberdashery and accessories; I'm sure we Dollman girls kept them in business.

The weekly comic cuts, together with the daily Adelaide Advertiser (owned and run by Keith Murdoch, father of Rupert) arrived in town via the steam train and Hall's bus. Pascoe's Newsagency was an important stop to collect comics on the due date. Once the comics were read, they were exchanged and collected. We did not get them regularly, as for a family of five they were expensive at three pence each!

My closest friend

My closest friend was Diana Dow. She had two brothers, Graham and Reg, who were about the same ages as Fuff and Peg. They lived four doors away up the hill on the corner of Ware Street and our parents were friends. We attended the same church and Graham Senior worked for Dad for a time so we did many things together. Throughout their friendship, my mother never called Mrs Dow by her Christian name Myrtle - or vice versa. Other close neighbours and friends were the Morgans, who had two younger girls.

Christmas, birthdays & holidays

Christmas, birthdays and school holidays were eagerly awaited events and unlike today, time dragged until the next special occasion. We all celebrated our birthdays with simple parties and attended those of friends who could afford them. Only special friends came, maybe up to eight or ten. The food usually consisted of bread and butter sprinkled with hundreds and thousands (a great favourite), sausage rolls and fairy cakes ... and of course jelly. Other fancy cakes were in the form of mushrooms, swans and cream horns depending on the prowess of the cook as all were homemade. If available, the cream-filled iced green frogs from Balfours in Adelaide and Cadbury's chocolate frogs made the party complete. Paper hats and sometimes balloons set the scene, and party games provided the entertainment. Hankies, chocolates, hair ribbons and inexpensive books were typical presents. We wore our party frocks and a wonderful time was had by all.

Christmas was usually spent at home with a hot midday dinner of roast duck or goose, and Christmas pudding (seeded with sterilised silver coins, threepences, sixpences and shillings) with custard and cream. We didn't much care for the pudding but liked a generous serving for the possibility of finding the coins. Of course the server ensured that each child got at least one coin.

On Christmas Eve, we all went shopping for Mum's last minute presents, and to view the Christmas trees and bunting the shopkeepers strung between the verandah posts in front of their shops. There was always a Father Christmas in Bences or Drew and Crewes, and the Salvation Army band played carols in the Rotunda in Market Square. After the shops closed we walked home, and with great excitement put out raspberry cordial and a plate of cherries for Father Christmas, and a carrot for the reindeer in front of the fireplace. Before going to bed, we also hung pillowcases for our presents at the bottom of our beds. Then followed a restless night as we tried to stay awake in the hope of catching a glimpse of the elusive Father Christmas. Mummy had to wait until well past midnight before creeping in to fill the waiting pillowcases. Next morning we sat on beds pulling out comics, sweets, knick-knacks, small toys and games, and one larger present (perhaps to be shared and possibly made by Dad) from our parents and perhaps Grandfather. It was rare to receive expensive presents as children do today, but we were all very excited and perfectly content with our gifts. I do recall Helen receiving a second-hand freshly painted bicycle, which she had seen and went back to the shop repeatedly to look at it. She nagged at Dad who eventually bought it, whether for Christmas or birthday, I do not know. None of the rest of us wanted one. When young Guy came along things were different and he received a scooter and a bicycle. Everyone spoiled him.

Holidays in Adelaide

The really special occasions were the school holidays, when we all bundled into the motor car and drove a hundred miles to Adelaide. As sections of the road were unmade, dust would seep into our cases tied on the luggage rack at the rear of the motor car.

At first when very young, we stayed with Grandfather at Walkerville. Auntie Kath and the two younger boys, Arthur and Firth, were still living at home. Dad who never stayed, as he could not leave 'the shop' (garage workshop), drove home the same day - another three hours alone. Quite probably, he sang without all the little girls forever chattering or playing in the backseat. We loved these visits as we were very spoiled by Auntie Kath. She showed us the sights of the big city with visits to the zoo, picnics in the Botanical Gardens, and trips by train to the hills and to Waterfall Gully; such wonderful adventures for little country girls. We rode the trams into the city where we shopped at the big city stores and ate cakes at Balfours.

Simple delights

The trams were the greatest thrill. When we lay in bed and heard the zing-zing as they were stopping, we knew we were in the city and we tingled with excitement. We loved to ride the trams and the tickets were a novelty. The tram used to make special stops so the conductor could alight and deposit the used ticket butts in our letterbox. Hearing the zing-zing, we would rush out to collect our treasures. I cannot imagine today that anyone would think of, or find the time to do such a thing, just to bring pleasure to little girls. We were thrilled to hear the postman's whistle when delivering the mail, a sound unknown to country children. Such small things brought great delight to us when we were young.

A gift of a penny was like receiving gold, long treasured and remembered - I have never forgotten how special the penny was that Uncle Harry gave me. One could buy an icecream with a penny, or keep it together with the memories of the kind person from whom it came.

Memories of Uncles Arthur and Firth, and Auntie Kath playing tennis on the court in the garden, the tame magpies, and the smell of the gas cooker come flooding back. Visiting old Great Auntie Jess, all shrouded in black, who lived in a home nearby was like seeing someone from centuries past.

8 Broadway, Glenelg

When I was about eight, Grandfather moved to 8 Broadway, Glenelg, just five houses from the Esplanade and a safe beach where he walked and swam daily until he was ninety. It was a large two-storey home with a long wide entrance hall, sitting room, dining room, kitchen, scullery, a big walk-in pantry for non-perishables, and five bedrooms, two of which had adjoining box rooms used for storage of travelling trunks and luggage. There was also an attic filled with exciting treasures.

We children were intrigued by the bell system on the kitchen wall, just like a stately home, with connections to various rooms. The bells were used from other rooms, particularly by Grandfather. At mealtimes, Auntie Kath or Grandfather rang the bell for the housekeeper in the kitchen.

The house had only one bathroom downstairs, which was usual, and we all seemed to manage even with nightly baths. A second toilet outside the back door, a common feature in Adelaide in those days, served for emergencies, the daily help and gardeners. A great attraction was the large terraced lawn in the back garden where we spent hours rolling down the slopes. Auntie Kath invited friends and cousins, threw parties and served us lunches and tea there. On hot summer nights, we slept on the lawn after she had ensured that we were protected from dampness and any nasty mosquitoes of the night.

Auntie Kath took us swimming and organised picnics on the beach. She must have spent every waking moment thinking of how to entertain us. Of course Mummy was there and helped too, but Auntie Kath was the mistress of the house and had Grandfather's money at her disposal. The cost of our entertainment was never an obstacle. She bought us clothes and as most things were charged, I expect she must have had an allowance for household expenses. Grandfather used to say, 'Kath does what she wants, you can't tell her anything.' And so he asked no questions.

The Ice-Man cometh

For many years, the household relied on an icebox for chilling foods and the iceman called daily with huge hessian-covered ice blocks piled on his cart. The iceman was another who spoiled us children. He would chip off pieces of ice into the hands of eager children, who would suck and savour the delicious coolness. Auntie Kath wanted a refrigerator; however Grandfather thought it quite unnecessary and had said 'No!' Undeterred, Auntie Kath bought one, and it was duly placed in the kitchen. Grandfather never went in the kitchen, as it was the domain of Elsie the housekeeper. Elsie was sworn to secrecy, and Grandfather's questions about the strange noises coming from the kitchen, which was next to the dining room, were warily passed over. Finally, his curiosity got the better of him and he ventured into the kitchen to find Kath's newest acquisition placed over the cool cellar, and producing the vibrating noise.

The secret Renault

I transgress to give another example of Kath's deception, which occurred many years later when she was in her mid-fifties. After years of catching buses and trams late at night and walking along the seafront from Jetty Road, she decided she wanted to be independent and so bought a car. It was a Renault purchased on time payment through Dad, the presence of which was unknown to Grandfather for some years. She would park it out on the street until he was safely indoors, and then roll it quietly down the hedge-lined drive to the garage at the back, another place he never visited. Her secret surfaced when some friend or relative happened to mention Kath's car to her bewildered father.

We all shared many adventures with Auntie Kath as she drove everywhere. Even my children when very small remember the car breaking down on East Terrace, and the experience of riding in the tow truck. On my last ride with her driving south of Adelaide, she lost her way and pulled off the highway. She then suddenly turned around to go back the way we had come, confusing all the following traffic. She had travelled the route often but this day she had come from a different direction. Despite having an unblemished driving record over forty years, doubtless at ninety plus, her eyesight was not as it should be for driving a car.

A chauffeur at our disposal

Grandfather worked as General Manager of the SA Brewery Co until he was ninety, and was blind for the last four of those years. Throughout this time and even after retirement, he had his own company car and uniformed chauffeur, who picked him up each morning and drove him home at night. Mac, as he was called, was also available each Saturday to take him and Kath to the races. For a time Grandfather was the Chairman of the SAJC (South Australian Jockey Club), a very prestigious position, and for years there was a race named after him.

The availability of Mac and the car extended to most members of the family, a privilege we all enjoyed when like royalty we travelled in a chauffeured car. Actually, we just accepted it as normal when staying with Grandfather. Mac worked in this position for at least thirty years, and was like a member of the family. He loved to tease us and delighted in calling Peg, 'Piggy'.

During my early teens when living with Grandfather, Auntie Kath enrolled me in a drama school in the city and Mac chauffeured me there too - on the way to the races I believe. Fuff too, when enrolled at Miss Mann's Business College in 1937 was dropped off in the mornings.

Summer holidays

From when I was about eight, Grandfather rented a large flat on the seafront for us during the summer holidays - usually at Semaphore. What wonderful days were spent swimming and building huge fortresses from the abundant piles of seaweed washed up with the tide. We had lunches and picnic teas under umbrellas to protect us from the hot afternoon sun. In those days, we also wore colourful beach pyjamas and hats. There were walks down the long jetty, the occasional camel ride on the beach and visits to the fun-park. For a time Auntie Jess was living at Carlton Flats, around the corner on Hart Street, and we loved to visit her. She introduced us to the novelty of nasturtium sandwiches, and showed how she had painted the interior walls of the house by applying, with a sponge, three coats of different pastel-coloured paints creating a lovely soft dappled effect. Back in Burra, Peg always the creative one promptly painted her room in this manner. In addition, there was the excitement of rides in the back of Uncle John's car, a two-seater sports car with an open air 'dickie seat' where the boot would normally be.

The summer Guy was born, Mummy stayed at home and Auntie Nora looked after us in Semaphore. Although we knew nothing about the facts of life, being told that the stork brought babies or that they were found under a cabbage was very hard for a five year old to comprehend! Auntie Jess came to tell us that when we went home there would be a surprise for us when we got home. One of us said 'Dinah has had pups' and Jess corrected her, 'You have a baby brother. Well what a surprise after four girls!' Auntie Kath always said my response was 'I suppose Mummy's tummy has gone all poof!' - indicating a collapsed tummy. We stayed longer to give Mum time with the new baby while we girls attended a nearby school for a few weeks.

What a charmed life we had thanks to Grandfather and Auntie Kath. Auntie Kath continued throughout her life to treat us as her own children, and I really believed that she thought we were. Until her death, she visited us all regularly, and was close to and loved by Errol and all our children.

One holiday Auntie Nora invited two of us to stay with her and our cousins Deidre and Cynthia at Port Lincoln on Eyre Peninsula. Uncle Bill Wincey was a geologist and away working with a mining company in New Guinea. Fuff and I were the lucky chosen ones, as I was closest to Cynthia in age, and Fuffy being very responsible was to look after me on the overnight boat trip. We embarked on the Minnipa from Port Adelaide, no doubt watched with much envy by Peg and Helen. Fuff recalls with much amusement that Mummy warned us to be very careful of what we ate on board in case of stomach upset and seasickness, and what did we eat - sardine sandwiches! When we pulled up at the wharf, I exclaimed, 'That looks like Mummy on the wharf', for to me Auntie Nora looked exactly like our mother.

The next few weeks were full of adventures, boat trips to nearby islands, picnics on the beach, and exploring the island. It was on these excursions the young Wincey girls, then aged eleven and seven, introduced us to the facts of life. Together with their friends, they gave demonstrations of intimacy to two bewildered, innocent Dollman girls. The young of Port Lincoln were certainly way ahead of us in Burra. We learnt more about the evolution of life through the breeding of silkworms, as the girls had a large shed where they showed us their fascinating life cycle. Breeding silkworms and spinning the silk was a favourite hobby for children in those days.

On Sundays after church, as was the Wincey's practice, we went to a local hotel for our Sunday dinner. This was a special occasion for us, as it was very formal.

On other short holidays, we drove over to Winkie, near Berri on the River Murray, where Uncle Harry had a fruit block. It was one of those, which were given to ex-serviceman after World War I. We eagerly anticipated these visits for the variety of fruits waiting to be picked and consumed: huge navel oranges, grapes, peaches, nectarines and apricots. The size and flavour of these is still not surpassed today. Each season Uncle Harry used to ship to us by road and train, a crate of his delicious navel oranges.

Beds were in short supply in Winkie and we used to love sleeping two in a bed, top to tail. At that time there were three Bryant children, twins Joan and Marie, a little older than I was, and Ross a little younger. Kevin came many years later.

Schooling

At the time, Fuff and Peg were approaching school age, and Mum who had been a teacher herself became interested in their schooling. Together with other young mothers in the parish, she was instrumental in establishing a small church school in St Mary's Sunday School. Peg and Fuff attended until the school closed - they were in Grades VI and VII respectively.

As Fuff needed some cosmetic dental work (braces), she went to Adelaide to live with Grandfather and attend The Wilderness School, a private school for girls for a year. Peg went on to the Burra High School, but also joined Fuff for three months at The Wilderness, as Fuff was lonely! Of course, Grandfather Bryant footed all the bills and Kath was happy having her two eldest nieces with her. On the girls return to Burra, they attended the High School, where Helen and I were, by then, in the Primary School.

Burra Model School

The Burra Model School is a magnificent building. It was built of local stone by a local firm, Sara & Dunstan, at a cost of less than 14,000 pounds, and opened in 1878 as a primary school. The town mine had closed a few months before, and while the school could accommodate 800 pupils, it enrolled fewer than 400 on opening day. In 1913, the High school opened in the west wing of the building with 35 pupils. The building still stands today, in its fine setting on the hill between Burra and Burra North.

Mum was not keen to relinquish her youngest daughter to the public system at the usual age, and decided instead to keep her at home, where she could tutor her. June could already keep pace with Helen in reading and writing, and Mum believed June should go straight into Grade II. However, this was not to be, as Miss Pearce ruled the roost in the lower grades where she had taught for as long as anyone could remember.

I was very anxious to start school, as I loved learning. I made friends easily and two of the other three Junes in the class, June Bourman and June Culpin were my closest friends for many years - unfortunately, we lost touch over the years. I had no difficulty with my studies and competed successfully with the other two Junes reaching 'top of the class'.

Miss Pearce was the proverbial spinster teacher-tyrant, though she was praised in the district as a fine teacher. I can only wonder at the damage done to shy, slow students in her charge. She went around the room, striking with her pencil the knuckles of luckless and frightened little pupils, who were always fearful of an attack. I remember well the times she stood over one very tall, shy, slow-speaking farm boy in the corner, and calling him every name related to dull, dumb, dim-witted, simpleton that she knew. I forever felt sorry for that poor boy and others whom she abused. So much so that at the Back to School Dinner during the town's 150th Anniversary celebrations, that when people praised Miss Pearce (long since dead) for her fine teaching, I could not hold back and stood up and told of what I had witnessed and my opinion of this 'fine' teacher. Students who achieved results did so, not because of her, but because they were bright and she left them alone, or they were outgoing and left untouched by her bullying. That same boy attended the dinner, and almost seventy years on was still slow speaking, and an even taller farmer.

It was very rare for us to have lunch at school, as Mummy always cooked a hot dinner in the middle of the day. After housework, this was a major feat for her in the middle of the day, and the return trip home for us meant we were often rushing to get back to school. Children from poorer families usually took bread and jam sandwiches, or bought mouth-watering Cornish pasties that were sold each lunchtime at the school gate. These were thrippence (three pence) each and buns were tuppence (two pence). We envied these children with their delicious pasties and pies. On the occasional Monday washdays, our wishes were granted and we were allowed to buy lunch.

Schooling

Our mother strongly believed in a sustaining hot meal each day, and also that hot bread or toast could not be properly digested. Our toast was always cold, much to the humour of the Dow boys who loved to ridicule our actions. On wet days, Dad drove us each way to school. In all his working life, he never walked the short distance to work as he always had something pressing to do and the car was there. However once at work he ran around from early morning till night.

Going to and from school was an adventure. It was about a twenty-minute walk, and half an hour if one dawdled. We went via Market Square through the shopping and business area, and then on to cross Burra Creek. Here we had two choices, to take the swaying suspension bridge, which was longer but only necessary if the creek had water, or to cut through the creek bed, which was much shorter. We loved the sway of the bridge, and always used it when coming home or when not rushed.

We enjoyed our walk to school and the creek was a playground for the wayward child. It was where my friends and I often lingered on our return home, playing and talking among the trees. I once recall arriving home far too late: it was after six o'clock. Dad was waiting at the back door with his threatening strap in hand and telling me to go inside, and I was hesitating fearing the strap on my legs. Of course, it was more threat than punishment and a way of stressing the importance of obeying our parents. The walking path was open and cleared but the banks elsewhere had many hiding places and it was no place for small girls to play. Not to mention the worry our parents would have gone through when we were not home from school.

Our parents were always very protective. They always had to know where we were going. Even in our late teens, we had to ask their permission and they then stipulated the time of our return. Our mother did not approve of our going out two nights running. Balls and dances were normally held on a Friday night and Saturday was the weekly night for the pictures, so if we went to the former we could not go to the latter! Although Fuff said the rules were less strict when Helen and I came along, claiming that 'You got away with more'.

Our school days were comparatively happy and as I continued to do well I had no problems. I do remember one embarrassing moment. When entering Mrs White's Grade IV class, by way of introduction, she told the class that my father had a beautiful singing voice and that doubtless I did too, and invited me to demonstrate. I was so embarrassed about my lack of talent I wanted to sink through the floor, but she persisted and somehow I struggled through. The whole incident remains an unforgettable memory of my school days. I recall also an instance when I did not want to go to school, and stayed in bed pretending to be sick. However my mother insisted I go, and by then as I was late and frightened of facing Mrs White I dawdled on the way; lingering in the creek bed, watching ants as they scurried about their daily chores, and then hiding behind trees, not wanting to be seen as I came up the hill to the school. I waited until after recess to join the rest of the class, hoping that I had not been missed ... but horror of horrors, Mrs White had spotted me and did all in her power to ridicule me as a truant. She seemed to delight in tormenting her pupils. It was unfair as I was a good student, and she attended our church and was a friend of our parents.

Before school we lined up in the schoolyard and with the flag raised to the accompaniment of the school band, we sang the National Anthem - God Save the King. On special occasions, we sang other patriotic songs like God Bless the Prince of Wales and The Song of Australia. After singing, we did exercises, which were necessary to combat the cold winters. All classrooms had wood fires, which were the responsibility of the boy wood monitor. In summer, the solid stonewalls assisted in keeping out the heat, and fortunately, the worst heat was in the summer holidays.

Common sports played were netball, tennis, football, cricket, vigoro (a form of cricket for girls) and athletics.

Woodlands CEGGS

When I was aged twelve and in Grade VI, I developed rheumatic fever. A specialist in Adelaide, Dr Begg, detected a heart murmur and

SCHOOLING

recommended that I would improve if I could get away from the dampness and cold of Burra. And so, midway through the year, Auntie Kath organised that I should live at 8 Broadway, Glenelg, and attend Woodlands - a nearby private school for girls. I don't know how much say Grandfather had in the decision, but he paid the school fees. Once again, Auntie Kath had the status of de facto mother of a daughter at an exclusive private school, a role that she filled for three and a half years with caring dedication.

These years were happy though somewhat tumultuous. For some inexplicable reason to me and everyone else at the time, I was forever in trouble. Now years later, I have worked out a possible explanation for my behaviour. My first day was the start of the winter term midway through the year, and so I received more than the usual attention. I was bombarded with questions from the daughters of Adelaide's lawyers, doctors, and dentists, with their exotic and hyphenated names - there were certainly no ordinary Jones or Smiths! Being from the country, it was assumed my Daddy must surely be a station owner.

This was rather a case of my inferiority complex, and a form of reverse snobbery as these girls were all very friendly. Subconsciously I believe I set out to test the rules and to gain a small reputation. This was quite unnecessary, as by the end of the year, I had topped the class - even in French, which the others had studied for some years. My misdemeanours were very mild compared to today, mostly so small I cannot remember. I was a target for accepting dares like climbing up the forbidden water tower and playing tricks on those teachers easily confused. As I always owned up, I was usually accused first. I did gain a reputation for honesty. In fact, one of my best memories is when I was a boarder and wanted the necessary permission to leave the 'prep' room. After finishing my homework I approached the dreaded Senior English/ Latin Mistress, Miss Baddams (later headmistress), to test me as was customary. To my amazement, she said, 'I don't have to test you June as I know that when you say you have done something, you have done it.' To my knowledge, she never failed to test anyone else.

Miss Glover my English teacher was responsible for the annual school magazine and not so trusting as 'Badds'. One year I wrote a poem of which I was quite proud. After the magazine came out she approached me and said, 'June, I did not include your poem as it was so good I thought you must have copied it.' She had not even asked me about it before making her judgement, and this disappointed me greatly as I was her top English student.

Herewith the poem:

Tramp Tramp Tramp
Marching forth to fame
Those valiant hearts
To carry on the name
O' a nation that was born
And e'er more shall be
The hearts and souls of men
Who venture forth for thee

Tramp Tramp Tramp
That sound is heard no more
But for the memories
Of those left behind
Whose bitter hearts are sore

Dear Auntie Kath had more faith in my literary ability, when at a tender age she took me and my book of writings (including 'And She Smiled') off to meet the editor of The Adelaide Advertiser. Overall, the poems were probably pretty pathetic, but I was very young. No doubt, he said to continue my brilliant work and that it was not yet ready for publishing. I must say Auntie Kath was wonderful in encouraging us all in everything we aspired to. Many years later, I enrolled in an Alan Marshall (writer and cartoonist) writing course by correspondence, but am ashamed to say I did not submit one article. I think maybe having to go to the garage to use the typewriter, and a talent for forever making spelling and other errors put me off. Besides, I had other priorities, playing basketball, tennis and badminton, and boyfriends

I made many friends and sailed successfully through my studies. The only mar on those days was the mounting black disorder marks, which seemed to keep pace with my scholastic marks. This caused much anguish to Auntie Kath and Grandfather, not to mention me. Each night I earnestly prayed to God to let me be good, and please not to get any more disorder marks. No matter how much I prayed the prefects and especially the sub-prefects, revelling in their power, followed me around and doled them out willy-nilly. Finally, when one point away from the permitted thirty (before facing the School Board), I was summoned to the office of 'Milly' the headmistress. Miss Millington's threats, God, or the start of a new year and a clean slate saved me from expulsion ... or maybe I left school that year. After I had left school, one young teacher who unknowingly had borne the brunt of my harmless jokes was speaking to one of my friends and remarked, 'You know, I always liked June, she was a lot of fun.'

I was dux at the end of my second year, and it was recommended that together with two other girls we miss Sub-Intermediate. We were to go straight into Intermediate, which concluded with a statewide examination, equivalent to Year 10 nowadays. I continued to do well but as it turned out it was quite a challenge.

Although most of my close friends were now in a class behind me, we continued to see a lot of each other as many lived in Glenelg. I also made many new friends, and Auntie Kath always encouraged me to invite them to stay for the weekend. I in turn was invited to stay at their homes. One of my best friends was Betty Gardner, who lived in Glenunga and travelled by tram to and from school. Tram travel was a great way for girls and boys from the private schools to make each other's acquaintance. She disclosed that she had caught the eye of a St

Peter's boy, and on investigation, I discovered that it was Reg Dow originally from Burra. Mrs Dow, Graham, Reg and Diana, had moved to the city and the children were attending private schools. Betty was delighted to hear that I knew the family thereby enabling her to get to know Reg better, which she did accompanying him to school dances and inviting him to her parties and dances. I recall the many visits to their lovely home and one party in particular when Auntie Kath made me my first long dress. It was a dream of white chiffon with coloured ribbon bordering the full skirt, neckline and sleeves, a gown fit for a princess, a fifteen-year-old princess!

Betty and sister Averil had a 'Nanny', who lived with them and was like a member of the family as she had been Mrs Gardner's nanny when a child. Betty and I were special friends, and she spent several holidays in Burra. She had an aunt who lived two doors away on our street and with her husband ran the local grocery store. My recollection is that during those holidays most of our time was spent following the local boys around, and vice versa. Students who attended private schools were fancied more by the locals of the opposite sex. Betty seemed to attract more than her share of males, and consequently her friends benefited too! Sadly, Betty contracted tuberculosis before she was twenty and died a few years later – she had only just married.

Another special friend was Maxine Fraser (Frizzy), who lived just around the corner from School. She was an only child and although they were apparently not wealthy, was spoilt in that she had everything before anyone else, new bicycle, tennis racquet, watch and always-new clothes. The latter were not wasted, as was clearly evident when holidaying at our home in Burra. Every day she had five different changes of clothes: one set when she got up in the morning, another after breakfast when we went to meet friends or to the shops, a third for lunch, then to go out in the afternoon and the last in the evening. I had to make do with three changes or less! Our outings were usually no more than walking, exploring the town, meeting friends etc. Although we were keen tennis players and Maxine had coaching at Memorial Drive, I do not recall tennis as part of our holiday pursuits.

There was much to see in Burra and many boys; like Betty, Maxine attracted them like a magnet.

On weekends in Glenelg, my friends went to the beach, into the city, to the shops or to the pictures. Those who had bikes either donkeyed me around, or I borrowed one and joined them on rides.

At the end of my last year, Grandfather was not at all well and no doubt was tired of my disruption to the household. Despite it being a large home, there was only one bathroom and at times, he was heard to call out 'Is that girl still in there?' He was not demonstrative and was very kind and loving to all his family. Our greeting was always a kiss on top of his almost bald patch. Mum told us his personality changed after the premature death of his beloved Katie (wife), who died when my mother was twenty.

With Grandfather now in his nineties it was decided that I should board. I enjoyed this period of my life very much. My group's dormitory was a large balcony, with canvas blinds on two sides that were drawn at night. I adjusted to rising at six in the extreme cold and to two-minute showers. We each had a small cubicle where we dressed and kept our possessions. I was able to realise the dream of every young girl reading of boarding school life, even to 'midnight picnics', which I organised. My mother willingly obliged and sent a big box of food by train. At the appointed time and place, we gathered and disposed of the goodies. Once a prefect discovered us but I do not recall the punishment, doubtless it was more disorder marks.

I broke more rules by putting on a school hat and gloves during after school sports and riding out of the school grounds on the back of Maxine's bike to her home. Such a petty thing, but in those days for boarders to leave the grounds without permission was a strict breach of school rules.

At night we always dressed for dinner, and in summer were required to have at least two frocks made from Liberty Swiss lawn cotton. It can still be bought from the famous Liberty store in London and is available from their shops around the world - including Sydney.

We could choose our own style to be made in any of the myriad of beautiful floral materials. To view their range is an absolute joy. In winter, the requirement was a velvet dress, more often with a lace collar. These frocks were worn one night a week (I do not remember which night) and on special occasions. The girls all dressed in the many rich velvet colours presented an exotic picture on these nights.

Sunday, dressed in school uniform we marched in crocodile file to the nearby St Peter's Church for morning service. Afterwards we were free to leave for an outing under the supervision of a relative or friend, who had to seek permission in advance. Twice during each term, full boarders (as opposed to weekly boarders, who went home every weekend) were able to have a weekend away with friends, provided it was pre-arranged by the hostess and the school.

Because I had a heart murmur, the specialist had advised against playing sports that involved running. The most popular winter sport hockey was ruled out, so I played basketball (now netball) and tennis in the summer. I excelled at basketball and when I was still fourteen I made the A Grade team, which was a great feat as all the other team members were sixteen or seventeen years old. I was selected to play defence, though was a good goalie too.

At Woodlands I first became interested in art, and the art teacher encouraged me in sketching and pottery, both of which I took up later in life. The art room was in a small cottage on the edge of the grounds. From near here my friends and I made an exciting discovery, which gave us many hours of pleasure. Hidden amongst the trees, just inside a private property there was a dolls house, fully furnished and large enough for several young girls to gather. It became our clubhouse, and there we held meetings into serious matters such as an investigation into puberty, when we sat around counting our pubic hairs! I don't recall if there was a prize!

SCHOOLING

Burra High School

I returned to Burra and started my Intermediate a year early. I only passed English of the nine subjects: English, Latin, French, German, Geography, History, Biology, Math I and Math II. Considering my excellent academic record, I am surprised that the school did not request a review of my papers, but perhaps as I had left the school they did not bother. Obviously I had not been ready to move up a grade, but I was disappointed as my friend Nadine Sparrow ('Spoggy') who had moved up with me, was not as good a student and had gained eight passes. As time later showed, I could not cope with external examinations in an unfamiliar environment and strange conditions. In Adelaide we rose early and travelled on foot and tram into the city, where the examinations were held in the huge army drill hall. Hundreds of students crowded into the hot, non air-conditioned hall in temperatures of 100 °Fahrenheit. As I suffered enormously from nervousness, it was not a good combination. Unlike today, no concessions were made for ill health or bereavement.

When I repeated the Intermediate Certificate at Burra High, Mr Eason the headmaster, encouraged me to tackle new subjects. He said that subjects such as typing, bookkeeping and shorthand would be useful. Three new additional subjects proved too much on top of five, and I was forced to drop two when others suffered. The result was that I did not pass my best subject, Maths. Mr Eason contacted the Examination Board, as I was his top student, but the mark was confirmed and once again, I failed, passing four subjects out of the required five!

My final year, I repeated a couple of my best subjects and four Leaving Certificate subjects, passing Intermediate and Leaving English and Geography - one short of the required three. I did not expect to pass Latin as my teacher chatted each lesson about everything other than Latin. One day she was fascinated by the appearance of a mouse, which thereon remained the main topic of every lesson. Ironically, I did not even learn the Latin word for mouse. In the Burra district, Leaving and Intermediate examinations were held together in the Institute - our

Town Hall. Leaving examinations were an hour longer than Intermediate and as I was the only one sitting Latin, I was left alone in the room after the other students left. The supervisor, the Catholic priest, came and stood behind me and asked me questions about whether I was having difficulties. I was too shocked and dumbfounded to respond, and he then answered sections of the paper and proceeded to translate the main and most difficult of all translations. I had never cheated and was appalled by his behaviour, especially as a priest. I was very upset and so confused that I could not remember anything he said, but the worst part was that I was an absolute wreck for the remainder of the time. I kept thinking what would he have done for me had I been of his faith! I was actually relieved when I failed, confirming that I had not benefited from his assistance.

I wanted to report him but who would believe a seventeen-year-old Protestant girl accusing a much-respected Catholic priest. He remained in the district for many years and I was plagued forever with thoughts of his continuing with such betrayals of trust.

Despite my failures, I was Dux of the school in that, my final year!

At High School, as my old friends had left school at age fifteen, I made new friends. My two special ones were Audrey Bowen ('Bunny') and Diana Davies. Audrey was doing Leaving, and Di I knew from our Church. My sister Helen and I hung around with Di and her older sister Joan; we were inseparable. We all practised for the church choir together, as well as going to dances and films. If someone had a boyfriend, the rest of us tagged along.

The Davies girls went out a lot more than we did, as Mrs Davies was much more lenient than our mother. When they came home in the early hours of the morning after a dance, 'Mrs D' would greet them at the door and point to the clock - no threats or reprimand! We were very envious. If we did likewise, we were told the house rules, and that if we did not like it we could leave. We had no money of our own, no place to go, and besides we did not want to leave our home and parents.

The War Years

On the 1st September 1939, Germany invaded Poland, and two days later Britain and France declared war on Germany. Australia, as a member of the British Empire was also at war. That was the year I entered Woodlands.

Young men were called up to serve their country, but having no brothers who were old enough our family was spared. Peg though, later joined the army and served in Australia. As a family we were not affected by any immediate tragedy, but we knew many who were - one family losing all four sons. Apart from loss of life, Australia was relatively unscathed.

Our war effort

Our early war effort consisted of entertaining our local boys when they came home on leave from training elsewhere in Australia. I was not really involved in this, as when war broke out I was thirteen and still at Woodlands. However when home on holidays I remember the singing around the piano, and the parties Fuff and Peg had to farewell their friends before they departed for service overseas. Then followed the baking of fruitcakes and packing of food parcels wrapped and stitched up in canvas, and the knitting of woollen scarves, balaclavas, mittens and socks needed for extra warmth and comfort.

Women knitted frantically night and day, whenever and wherever we were. We could not sit without knitting in our hands, even in the dark at the pictures. Knitting was very much a part of women's lives in those days. We all made many jumpers, and some of us even made dresses, mine being an attractive sage-green bouclé. My friend June Bourman was an obsessive knitter. In winter, she rose at five and started knitting while sitting by the wood stove, until it was time for breakfast and work. I was shocked when I went to live in Canada ten years later to find that nobody knitted, nor did they wear woollens. Buildings were so well heated; light garments were worn indoors and heavy overcoats or furs when outdoors. Nylon materials had replaced woollens.

After the fall of Singapore and as the Japanese drew closer to our shores the threat of an attack on Australia took on some reality. To most of us in the south, we still felt far removed from any danger and it seemed a bit ludicrous to set up spotting posts as the government had requested, but all Australia answered the call. Twenty-four hours a day two persons manned the post, working their shifts and diligently watching the skies for enemy planes. Our post was organised by Mrs Dulcie Richardson, an English lady whose husband sent her to Australia with their two children for the duration of the war. She first lived in Broadway, Glenelg, where Auntie Kath befriended her and so came to Burra as a result.

Until the Japanese bombed Darwin on 19th February 1942, we in the rest of the country did not realise just how vulnerable we were, nor did we know the severity of the surprise attack and the number of enemy planes heading south. Similarly, it was many years before Australians were told that the Japanese had evaded detection, and had managed to come right into Sydney Harbour. During the war there was tight security on such releases. As well, trenches were dug and arrangements made for safe haven in case of attack. Many of us had our cellars, and it was by the grace of God that they were never used.

Auntie Nora also came to Burra for a short time, and rented a house across the road from us. It had the only swimming pool in the town, which provided plenty of fun for us too.

Much time was spent raising funds for the Red Cross, including concerts, which toured the district and outlying towns. Our family and friends were all involved in one way or another. We had many excellent singers, young and old who formed a choir and sang solo and duets. Nell Pearce, a well-known soprano, sang many duets with Dad, as did Mavis Halliday. Joan Davies had won some talent quests as a popular singer and Helen sang songs from light operettas. I loved to hear her singing 'I'll Gather Lilacs' from The Merry Widow and I always think of her when I hear it. Helen did learn singing for a short time, travelling each week by train to Adelaide for her lessons. She was always very nervous and never sang enough in public to overcome it.

Rae Corry, the young wife of a local teacher, was very talented and taught a small group of eight girls to dance. We performed together, high kicking and tap-dancing in formation, a combination of The Rockets and marching girls on a lesser scale. Rae did all the choreography and designed our various costumes. We were quite professional and well received. There were numerous skits, Mr Rosman was an accomplished comedian and Dad was the popular compere, although Helen and I used to cringe at some of his shaggy dog stories. I guess we missed the point as the audience showed more appreciation; however, we burst with pride whenever he sang. Sadly we have no recording of his voice, as recording machines were unavailable to us, or we had not heard of them. Peg did pay for him to go to a recording studio in Adelaide, but unfortunately, he never took advantage of it. His numerous trips to Adelaide were always on business, and as it was still a two and half hour trip each way, he was always in a hurry.

Our nightly concert trips to the country were always a lot of fun. Generally, we all loaded into Teddy Lehman's bus (Teddy had taken over from Alec Bevan), but I suppose some went by car. We left home about six in the evening and got home in the small hours of the morning. It was work as usual the next day. During the interval, the country folk provided a sumptuous supper as only countrywomen can.

Other fund-raising efforts were the dances and balls, and any person who grew up in the country in those days will remember them with much fondness. It was the way young people met, and most romances blossomed in the dance hall before leading to marriage. In the smaller communities young and old participated, dancing, watching, preparing supper, or playing in the band. The girls sat around the room waiting to be asked to dance while the men gathered at the door and eyed off the girls. Some went out for a smoke or a sly drink, which were not to be consumed within a hundred yards of the hall.

Sometimes the girls snuck out for a nip of sherry or red wine, always known as plonk no matter how good, as it often was. Of course, the real intention of the boys was hoping for a bit of fondling, or more depending upon the girl. The 'fast' girls were well known and pursued, but girls whom they fancied were also targets. The boys with cars were popular among the girls, who hoped to be driven home followed by a kiss and a cuddle but no more. Most of us were so innocent that we had no idea of the joys of sex. Besides, our biggest fear was falling pregnant, which would have made us instant outcasts and embarrassed our families. In general, pregnant girls moved away to a home and to have the baby where it was adopted out. It was very sad, as many nice trusting girls were taken advantage of and public opinion was that the girls were to blame for being too 'easy'.

Boys, boys, boys!

During the war, the soldiers and airmen stationed nearby regularly came to our dances, and while many romances started, often they did not continue as the men were not around for long. We younger ones became friendly with some of the younger soldiers. We girls in our mid and late teens became the unofficial welcoming committee headed by Joan, Helen, Diana and June.

Joan and Diana were both very tall and glamorous and were magnets to the troops. Joan was slim with long blonde hair and in fact won the South Australian section of the Pix Magazine Girl of the Year. She would drape her slim body over a post in front of our garage, which was on the opposite corner to the army store. We had many photos of Joan with her long blonde hair flowing over one shoulder in a seductive pose that inevitably achieved the right response. Diana when aged fourteen was five feet eleven and with her lovely long auburn hair was always judged to be years older. Those two girls were true assets to our cause, and so we met many young soldiers who were anxious to give us their names and addresses.

Sometimes the convoys only stopped for refuelling when we would hastily scribble our names and addresses on the sides of the trucks.

Following this we would receive letters often with photographs enclosed and so the start of many friendships by correspondence, and at times future meetings. Joan met the man she married, after he came to Burra to meet her after a long correspondence. More than fifty years later, until his death, they were still happily married.

Writing to boys we knew in the forces (and many we didn't), kept most of us occupied. Many army convoys stopped in the town on their way north to the Northern Territory. There was a staging camp at Peterborough about forty miles north of Burra, and also an Air Force training station nearby. There were also half-a-dozen or so soldiers stationed in the town at an army store. When they moved on, others replaced them and we became friendly with many of them.

Fuff became friendly with Charlie Biggs, and he and his friends were entertained in our home. Although he was engaged, they kept in touch throughout and long after the war. The friendship continued with him and his wife in Adelaide, until they passed away.

I met a Bob Tye who was very keen and we corresponded for a time. Through him, I met Paul Danslow, who came to a dance and believing that I was Bob's girl, told me about his complicated love life saying that he had confessed his love to about three girls who insisted he prove it by getting engaged. They all lived in different states. He was only eighteen, as was I, so I doubt he had given them rings - only promises to marry. On learning that I was not Bob's girl, he became interested in me. When he moved away, we corresponded and met in Adelaide and other places until well after the war. He was not handsome, but very charismatic, generous and lots of fun. Though I liked him a lot and he always insisted he loved me, I never fell for it.

For a time I corresponded with a Bruce Nicholson from Melbourne, but sadly he was among troops lost when their boat was attacked and sank somewhere off New Guinea. One of his friends wrote to tell me but I never heard any further details. He was only nineteen and very handsome as portrayed in his photograph, which I still have. It seemed sacrilegious to throw it away.

I join the workforce

When I finished school, Dad was approached by the local manager of the Bank of Australasia (now the ANZ Bank) with the view to my joining their staff. Before the war, banks never employed females, but as most male staff were in the forces, young single girls were to be employed until the men returned.

In those days together with doctors, lawyers and the like, bank officers and stock agents were the plum jobs, and so I became an employee of that bank for the duration of the war. A year or so later, I was approached again, as many of the former staff either did not return or moved on to other professions. I was a ledger keeper and occasionally a relief lunchtime teller - a real breakthrough as telling was the sole domain of the male. In those days as there were no machines, all was done by hand and head. Though I enjoyed working with figures and weekly balancing of all accounts in pounds, shillings and pence, it was indeed a challenge, as we had to balance each day to the exact penny and could not go home until we did.

Weekly balances of all books could result in late departures, and the wee hours were not unknown when all staff would assist those who could not find that elusive penny. A long-time accountant, 'Ponty' (Frank Pontifex), was an absolute whiz with figures and knew all sorts of short cuts and idiosyncrasies of handling currency, as does Errol who also has worked in a bank. Ponty liked his drink, and during balance would go off to the hotel for added sustenance. His lovely wife put up with this excessive drinking. I can't imagine what she thought of his thrice-annual gifts of silk stockings purchased by one of the female bank staff for Christmas, Birthday and Mother's Day alike.

Incidentally, in 1951 after his arrival in Canada, Errol sent me a very special gift of six pairs of American pantyhose. In those early days, the nylon lasted forever, no runs or holes - unlike those of today. After years of mending silk and lisle stockings, nylons were a girl's best friend.

The exact practice of balancing was so unlike my experience a few years later when working in The Bank of Nova Scotia in Canada. Balancing was not taken too seriously, especially by the tellers who had much difficulty even with the decimal system and had an 'unders and overs' book. The ledger-keepers of the new-fangled machines (to my Australian eyes) had not a clue as to how they worked after they punched in the cheques. They had more difficulty in balancing, and therefore I was much sought after. To my amazement, the bank manager even reached for an adding machine to total a few small cheques before approving an overdraft on an account.

Weekends in Adelaide

In the latter part of the war when we were all working, we would take the train to Adelaide on holiday weekends. Two large suitcases would accompany each of us, which were filled with enough clothes for a month's stay. On arrival, we lugged the cases across the road to The Grosvenor Hotel, a very popular unlicensed hotel for families and country people because of its reputation and proximity to the railway station. The Grosvenor is now much more expensive and probably licensed, but in our day was very reasonable for our slim pockets.

Also on North Terrace and close by was the best hotel in Adelaide, The South Australian (now replaced) where Grandfather sometimes dined. He also regularly dined at the Imperial Hotel on King William Street. It was owned by the Brewery as were many hotels in Adelaide and the country towns of South Australia. Once when living in Glenelg, friends and I were passing by the Broadway Hotel as a truck was unloading barrels of beer. When one fell to the ground, one of the brewery employees remarked 'Wouldn't want old G.B. to see that.' I expect that he knew George Bryant lived on Broadway but he would have had no idea that GB's granddaughter overheard him.

As all businesses opened on Saturday mornings, we all worked and our holiday weekends apart from Easter were very short. We did very little other than enjoy the hotel and just being in Adelaide. We often walked along the lovely lawns of the Torrens and took one of the boat rides. We met many Americans on leave who were anxious to have company. At least one once when the weather was hot and balmy, we spent the night on the lawns beside the Torrens; and once up a tree for fun and to catch the breeze.

For most of us, it was all pretty harmless. Though who knows what happened when friends snuck past the watchful eye of the night porter at the Grosvenor. Paul did this a few times but it was difficult to do much when sharing a room. We were anxious to guard our reputation. Fuff stayed in the hotel a few times to meet me, and was very alert to what Helen and I were up to. She was not sneaky but felt her responsibilities as our older sister and was protective ... and just as well!

It is amazing how values have changed. Despite being in our late teens, we were so happy and did not think we were missing out. A bit of petting satisfied us but perhaps not always the boys, though they generally respected us for rejecting their advances. It was one of these weekends when a young American soldier, with whom I had been corresponding, organised leave in Adelaide to meet me. Until then we only had photos of each other. One evening we took the train to Semaphore, where we walked along the beach and long jetty, and then sat on the sand watching the sunset. Despite my protests, that night I lost my virginity at the ripe age of eighteen. He was nineteen and could not believe that any girl could still be a virgin. I did not blame him or feel that I had been raped, as he said after a year in the Pacific with no available women, he had been waiting for this moment and had no idea that I would not consent. Around eleven we went to catch the train back to the city only to discover that they had stopped running. We had no choice but to start walking. After covering some miles, we were fortunately picked up by an Advertiser van driver returning from his delivery rounds of the early edition of the newspaper.

My sisters marry

During this period, Peg finished working locally as a telephonist, and after joining the Army was sent to camps near Alice Springs and

Katherine. It was here she met Tom Stevenson, married, and became pregnant. She returned home to us where she had her first child, David, and they remained with us till the war ended, when she and Tom moved to Melbourne.

After leaving school, Fuff worked for Dad in the office for a short time, and then in 1940 joined The National Bank. I remember her excitement at receiving her first pay cheque and not only paying Dad and Mum board, but also handing to Guy and me our first pocket money, threepence for Guy and sixpence for me. I don't recall for how long this weekly allowance continued, but it was a very generous offer from a nineteen-year-old girl whose pay would have been quite meagre. I have never forgotten this gift from my loving and thoughtful sister. No wonder Dad always thought the sun shone out of her!

Helen too worked for Dad for a while, and then moved on to Goldsborough Mort Stock and Station Agents. Later she nursed at The Adelaide Children's Hospital, which was her true vocation, as she loved children and always said she wanted five of her own.

When she married Reg Clark they in fact had seven; but lost one of their first-born twins, Peter, at a few days old, and then Guy their third child in his second year. Poor Helen had a difficult time as their youngest child Diana was born with a congenital 'hole in the heart', and underwent a number of worrying, though successful, operations. Helen herself suffered from breast cancer and a mastectomy, and five years later, cancer of the stomach. She died shortly after the last operation at the age of forty-eight. She deserved better as was always a bright and happy person, and loved by everyone. She was a wonderful, caring nurse, who suffered along with her young patients and especially so whenever they tragically passed on.

V-Day – the end of the War

One memorable weekend in Adelaide, we celebrated Victory Day, signified by Winston Churchill holding his fingers in the famous V sign and the end of the war in Europe. Australia rejoiced with the rest of the world though few had been far beyond South Australia or Victoria. Crowds gathered, cheering and shouting in Adelaide's streets, and I remember being held high on Paul's shoulders.

After the War

After the war, life in Burra was very full as everything returned to normal and the boys were welcomed home. Our concerts continued raising money for Red Cross and local charities. We had an occasional weekend and holiday in Adelaide with visits to Semaphore Beach and Glenelg. Joan married Ian and moved to Melbourne, and Diana went with her. (Fifty years passed before we met again at a Back to School weekend in Burra.) I saw more of my friend Audrey, in fact we became inseparable and spent hours talking at Sara's Corner about goodness knows what, before parting to go home.

Tennis clubs re-formed and our Kooringa team played inter-club Saturday matches with teams from Burra North, Clare and small hamlets in the district - Farrell Flat, Booborowie, Hanson and others. Those of us without cars went with the few men who had a vehicle. How we survived the hot summer days, I will never know, as temperatures soared into the nineties and over the century. Fuff has told me of a time when the temperature was 111 °Fahrenheit (42.5 °C), and she and a friend went to tennis and wondered why no-one else had turned up! Tennis was a summer game, not played all year round as it is today. Between matches we cooled off temporarily with a beer at the nearby local, which was not air-conditioned, and then it was back to the hot, often hard-tar court.

We played without hats or sunglasses, and many a Saturday I returned home with a splitting headache. I recall standing under the shower with the cold water pouring over my head, trying to ease the pain. Nevertheless, nothing deterred me from my Saturday game and the daily practices with Audrey and others. In winter night badminton replaced tennis, and it was basketball for girls (rising early for practice before work), and football for the boys.

On Saturday nights we usually went to the weekly showing of pictures, with or without a boyfriend. At first there was a newsreel, then a cartoon followed by one film, an interval, and then the feature film. No one who ever went to these country picture shows could forget the ritual of interval, when all and sundry rushed to the nearby cafe to get a hot crusty Cornish pasty lavished with tomato sauce. It was sheer bliss to feel the warmth seep into and through our bodies on winter nights. I do believe they were enjoyed just as much in summer, except on the very hottest of nights when icecream was a welcome replacement.

I presume a similar scenario took place all over Australia, as there was very little heating in public places and none at all during the war. At the bank on bitterly cold days, we often wore our overcoats and mittens inside, as we were not allowed to turn on the electric heaters. Pies and pasties were the only fast food available in my youth, and I have yet to meet an Australian who rejected them.

Dances, dresses and courtship

These dances continued for various causes and clubs, and were where 'girl met boy' and vice versa. It was often the start of a relationship that led to marriage in country districts. In Burra, only the Catholic Ball had debutantes, although later when I was too old it became quite fashionable - so I never 'came out'. However, balls were always a great occasion for dressing up. We wore beautiful long frocks and there was often The Belle of the Ball competition, which I won a few times.

Audrey's mother was a very clever seamstress and I had an excellent dressmaker in Burra North. I also made many of my own clothes with Mum's hand operated Wertheim sewing machine, including both one-piece and two-piece bathing costumes. For many years and well into my marriage I wanted to be a fashion designer. I taught myself to follow the patterns, and after completing a one-year night course in pattern design started to incorporate my own ideas. I was so keen on sewing I even made dresses for a neighbour. As I was self-taught, it was not easy but I had patience and perseverance on my side. Quite unlike Peg, who without any tutoring had an ability to design and cut out clothes without the aid of patterns. I still marvel at seeing her (aged seventeen), make my lovely white Communion dress, simply by laying out the material on the floor and proceeding to cut out a complicated eight piece flared skirt with button-down front bodice and short puff sleeves. She was so quick, working without hesitation.

Peg was an excellent cook, though had a very short temper. I remember at least one occasion when in the midst of making pastry or scones, someone upset her and she threw the mixture all over the kitchen. My reaction was that I could never do that knowing I would have to clean it all up, but she quietly set to and cleaned it up. She took great pride in her cooking and displayed her handiwork in the cookery section in the annual Burra Show, as did Fuff and Helen, while I entered various flower arrangements. We all had won prizes in some categories from time to time. Later when David was born, she decided she would enter again. I had never learned cooking at school (too menial a pursuit for young Woodlands ladies), and as the others in my family were good cooks, I had done very little myself. I decided that I would like to enter cream puffs, following Peg's recipe. And the result ... I was awarded first prize with Peg's cream puffs second. Needless to say, she was not impressed!

Until I was about twenty, I had had only short casual romances. There were no serious boyfriends, though Paul came and went frequently from my life, and maintained that he was. Ross Bryant, my cousin, kissed me once behind Grandfather's couch, after which I considered him my boyfriend for a year or so. However, the first boy who really kissed me was Ross Humphries after taking me home from a Burra High School dance. I was home on holidays from Woodlands and went with Helen to the dance. I often wondered what Helen thought about being the only one who did not go away to school. She must have felt very left out, but when schoolmates asked her why she didn't go she just said that she did not want to, which I am sure was not the case. Poor Helen missed out on many things.

My first long-term boyfriend was Don Christie, who was transferred to the Burra branch of Elder Smith & Co. Ltd, Stock and Station Agents. He worked with Reg Clarke who was going out with Bunny (Audrey), ('dating' was an American expression not yet in vogue in Australia), and as she and I went everywhere together, Don made up the foursome. I had always tagged along even when Bunny and Reg became engaged! She was excited about being engaged but had no serious thoughts of marriage. She was very attractive with ash-blonde hair and had no shortage of boyfriends. Reg was the first to propose. After a year or so, he eventually tired of waiting and turned his attention to Helen. Referring to her as 'Tubby', as she was a little overweight, he had always admired her saying constantly to Bunny 'Why can't you be more like Tubby?' Later Helen and Reg married.

As often happens in small towns, Don and I spent all our free time together, except Saturday afternoon when I played tennis and he football. Once, he took me in an Elders vehicle to Adelaide for the weekend to stay with his mother and sister. His father had previously died after contracting tetanus from a simple cut while working on their farm. We were friendly for more than a year until he was transferred to Saddleworth, a small town nearby. Not long after I heard that he became engaged to a local girl. I thought we were in love, as did my parents and friends, as he always seemed very devoted. It was just as well that nothing came of it, as he went to a farm in Lameroo where surely I would have been bored stiff.

I turned twenty-one around this time, and Mum and Peg organised a party in the local Army Drill Hall. Many of the presents were vases, sheets, towels and other things for a glory box, in fact a dowry, which most girls had started though I had never done so. Surprisingly, Junie Culpin gave me a Stuart Crystal vase, which I still have. She was very clever and beautiful, reminding me of Anna Neagle, the film star. She lived with her grandmother in a small cottage, and although we were good friends, I never knew anything about her family and always thought they were very poor.

There were quite a few families like this in Burra, poor with no fathers, or with fathers who worked as council labourers or as wood carriers. As long as I remember, Mrs Seaford came every Monday to do our washing. She was a hardworking, rough but kind soul, who swore like a trooper, always referring to the clothes as 'the buggers'. She lived in an old run-down cottage with her two children, both of whom were quite intelligent; Myrtle was a friend of Helen's and in the same class, while Bob was in my class. Both went on to successful jobs. Many other families had strange Eastern European names like Hirschausen, Borowski and Kaukoschke. The latter were Catholics so we did not know them well, but those that we did used poor English, and we thought of them as quite uneducated and looked down on them. The Catholics mostly went to the Convent School, and the girls had a habit of poking out their tongues at us. This did not endear us to them, but no doubt we deserved it. The more uncouth Protestant boys responded with the vulgar chant 'Catholic pigs smell like dogs, jump like frogs' etcetera. For us, correct grammar and table manners were very important and I am ashamed to say we judged everybody by our standards. We were not unkind but there certainly was a class system. Far too late I realised many of these people were immigrants from Europe after the First World War, or even earlier. I am now sorry that I did not know more about their backgrounds.

One did not delve into peoples' private lives - it was not done. They either were not encouraged, or were anxious to forget their former lives, but I imagine that it was more the former as we were very much an Anglo-Saxon society and in the main Protestant. South Australia had only free settlers and was the only State not to take in convicts. Strangely, Dad who had received an excellent education at a convent in Wilcannia had no time for Catholics, always saying that, 'They could not be trusted and that you could smell them coming.' Possibly, he was referring to the Irish, who were not noted for their cleanliness. Even more strange was that his very close friend Norman Pearce had Catholic in-laws, the Killicoats, with whom we were very friendly. This feeling of distrust was inherent in most Protestants and Grandfather was very upset when his eldest son Harry married a Catholic girl. Though Harry's wife Stella promised that the children would be brought up as Protestants, only their eldest son Ross was. At Grandfather's expense, he attended St Peter's College, a private

Anglican school in Adelaide, though ultimately too he married a Catholic girl!

As we moved into our twenties we got to know some of the Catholics girls, and despite their bad grammar they were very nice. However, we were very intrigued when they told us that they could do anything immoral, tell lies, steal, even have premarital sex, and that all would be forgiven at the confessional - no doubt the reason for Dad's distrust.

Helen by now was nursing in Adelaide, and as she missed the family, came home at every opportunity. She would arrive late on bus (now Ted Lehman's), from the train station. Sometimes it was only for one day and she would return early the following morning. We were often woken by the sound of the bus horn in the early hours; typically, Helen had not heard her alarm and was still fast asleep. The ever patient and kind Teddy waited outside while Helen threw on her clothes and joined him. For longer breaks she sometimes brought home a friend, which was nice, and once or twice I went to Adelaide and stayed in the nurses' quarters. This was tricky, as I had to sneak in without being detected. Overnight visitors were strictly prohibited.

The twice-daily train to Adelaide was very much a part of our lives. When we went as a family Dad took us in his car, otherwise we used the train. It was an enjoyable and friendly experience as we sat in carriages, four on each side, facing each other. Sometimes we met people we knew or made new friends. Except for the Broken Hill Express we stopped at all stations along the way, with a longer stop for refreshments at Riverton, where pies, pasties, sandwiches, cakes and drinks were available. To travel in or to simply observe and hear a steam train, is the most wonderful and indescribably thrilling experience. Later there was the Barwell Bull, a diesel train, so named after a premier and very new at the time.

Bunny was accepted for nursing training at The Royal Adelaide Hospital in early 1949, and like Helen lived in the nurses' quarters, which enabled girls to have some welcome independence away from home. She had plenty of admirers and was very anxious for me to meet the friend of her current boyfriend, whom she said I would like and would be my perfect match. The next holiday weekend I went to Adelaide, and on the Saturday, the four of us went to the Royal Adelaide Show. She was right, as Ron Gurney and I had a mutual attraction for each other. I was twenty-three and he twenty-nine and he said that he was ready to marry. I met his parents and sister and the romance developed over the next few months, mainly by telephone.

Some months later Mum was invited to Sydney to meet her three best friends from teacher training. She had not seen them for thirty years and paid for me to go along with her. We went by bus and stayed with one friend, and had a lovely time meeting up with all three. We did the sights of Sydney and visited The Blue Mountains where one managed a lovely old home as a boarding house. I saw my mother in a completely different light, like a young girl as they all joking and laughing, recalled their younger days. Like all children but in those days especially, we could not imagine our parents as ever being young. Returning to Adelaide I was amazed when my mother, in fun, threw a paper ball at the bus driver.

As we had done on the way over we had an overnight stop, this time at Echuca on the River Murray, Victoria. I had told Paul Danslow that we would be stopping off there and he arranged to come to Echuca for the night to see me, which was nice of him. When our bus arrived back in Adelaide, Mum went to stay with Auntie Kath, and I went to stay at the Royal Adelaide Hospital with Bunny. There was always a spare bed that belonged to someone on night duty, and as with Helen, I had to sneak in. Bunny remarked that as I would want to see Ron, she would ring him to arrange a meeting with him and another friend. I was somewhat suspicious when without hesitation, she dialled Ron's telephone number ... she obviously knew it by heart!

That evening when Ron and his friend arrived, he opened the car doors expecting me to get in the front beside him. For some reason, or because I suspected he and Bunny had been seeing each other, I jumped in the back seat with his friend. Bunny got in the front with

Ron and so that was the end of my romance with Ron. I must say that had our roles been reversed, Bunny would have got in the front, but I was less confident with men. Later Bunny asked why I had jumped in the back, and on being told the reason she confessed that she and Ron had been out together a few times, but had only gone on condition that he resume his friendship with me on my return. As obviously he preferred her to me, I was no longer interested.

The following Christmas they announced their engagement on Boxing Day, and were married in April with me as a bridesmaid! Her mother was furious, as Bunny had been so excited telling her that Ron and I were serious with each other, and yet she had blatantly taken him away. On top of that, she had the nerve to ask me to be her bridesmaid! My only concern was that her love for Ron might wane as they got serious.

Even more difficult for her, was that same December she had received a letter from a doctor friend who was about to return to Australia after serving with the occupation forces in Japan. He was looking forward to seeing her, continuing their relationship and implying a proposal. Bunny had confessed her love for him and had been corresponding with him for a year, yet she was to announce her engagement a few days before his return. The following year she did not return to nursing, but stayed home to prepare for her marriage. She expressed some hesitation; however, they did marry happily - and to this day still are.

For some time she was jealous of me, confessing that she felt Ron wished that he had married me. For the first few months after their wedding, they lived with his parents. It was not a happy arrangement as his mother repeatedly told her that he should have married me; she had only met me once and the comment was just pure spite. Even after we had lived overseas for some years, it was interesting that Bunny was not at all keen for Ron and me to meet up again! That is all in the past now, as we do keep in contact and meet when we are in Adelaide. Had I married Ron, no doubt I would have been content, but would not have had all the exciting adventures, married Errol, and most of all had our wonderful children.

By contrast, their way of life is not what I have would have wanted, and Audrey's interests are now quite different to mine. Her mother was quite genteel and had German migrant parents who lived in the Barossa Valley. When she fell pregnant to this supposedly 'unsuitable' man, her mother virtually cast her out from the family - or so Bunny told me years later.

My next serious boyfriend was Frank Storey who came from Wangaratta in Victoria. His father had been manager of The Bank of Australasia, and he worked for Goldsborough Mort before his transfer to Burra. For the next eighteen months all of my waking hours, as they had been with Don Christie, were spent with Frank; dancing, on visits to our home, at the pictures and long walks on hot summer and cold winter nights. Favourite walks were beyond Queen Street to the outskirts of Kooringa and to an old derelict flourmill, which I had not previously known existed, and over the hill toward the mine site and Burra North. We made many discoveries in our desire to be alone and together. Frank lived in a low building attached and belonging to the Commercial Hotel, where he had his meals. This building had two bedrooms and a bathroom, which were rented to single employees of Goldsborough's, all rather primitive but cosy and warm. I sometimes visited and although there was a side door and gate to Queen Street, we were frightened of being seen. Small towns are rife with gossip, which not only travels fast but is often misinterpreted and can ruin reputations. It is ridiculous when one thinks that we were both at least twenty-three. Don and Reg had lived on the second floor above Elder's office and they were even more careful of having visitors. Consequently, I went there only once or twice.

Sometime in early 1951 Auntie Kath and I travelled to Brisbane, by train as far as Sydney and then onwards the following day by ship. We stopped overnight at the YWCA that was convenient to Central Station, and visited two of her old friends from nursing days in Broken Hill. One friend, despite having an artificial leg since childhood, had not been deterred from undertaking the arduous profession of nursing. After leaving her flat in Kings Cross, we took a bus to the city where we attempted to find a taxi. This proved impossible as it was raining and a Friday. We started walking with hand luggage (I presume our cases had been forwarded direct to the ship), hoping to get a taxi on the way. In the end, we had to run towards Pyrmont docks where our ship was about to depart. While running across the old Pyrmont Bridge, I said to Auntie Kath, 'I am glad that it is you with me and not Mummy.' I did not recall ever having seen my mother run, as those were the days when it was unseemly for ladies, even the young and particularly once one was married. Auntie Kath ran all her life, maybe it was because she was a spinster until her seventies, or more likely, because she broke every golden rule. We reached the quay to find the gangway had been taken up, however not all was lost and we were hoisted aboard by crane, like baggage in a basket. After such a memorable departure, we arrived in Brisbane without further incident, in time to fulfil our duties as godmothers at the christening of Peg and Tom's daughter Susan (the twins, Jane and Rick came later). We stayed two weeks in a nearby hotel on the beachfront and spent our days with Peg and family before flying back to Adelaide. On the flight from Brisbane to Sydney, we had a clear view of the coastline and its long sandy beaches fringed with beautiful white surf. We could almost hear the crashing sound of the surf and I was struck by the sheer beauty of the coast, at that time totally undeveloped.

I must break here to tell a story from the First World War that illustrates just how unconventional Auntie Kath was. When serving in Alexandria, Egypt, she was invited by a sheik to visit his home. They went by train and she became very worried because it was a long journey, even more so when they arrived at his grand house where she was given a drink. Fearing that he might have an ulterior motive, she managed unobtrusively to 'slip' (in her words) the contents of her glass into a potted palm. Despite her concerns, after a pleasant meal she was delivered safely back to camp.

After The War

Around this time, Errol Burdon entered my life. In his early teens he had lived in Burra with his father, who was stationmaster, elder sister Rita and elder brother Ivor. A year younger than Fuff, Errol had known her at high school. Errol and a friend, Alan Walker, had carried home the schoolbooks of Fuff and her friend Jean Banks who lived nearby. The boys who lived in Burra North had bicycles and I remember Fuff making some lame excuse to Mum that it was too hot to do their homework inside, so they could study on the front verandah and chat to the two boys hanging over their bikes on the street. With the exception of those who attended our church, we generally did not know much about the families who lived in Burra North.

Many years later Errol's father returned to Burra, as did Ivor, his wife Blanche and their two little children, Helen and Peter (Margaret arrived later). Ivor was senior teacher at the high school. They lived four doors away and I played tennis with Ivor and Blanche. When visiting his father and Ivor, Errol asked me out but as I had a boyfriend I refused. On the second occasion, however I was very tempted, but again I declined. Mum and Dad both agreed that it might harm my relationship with Frank.

In the interim Errol obviously had spoken to Ivor who told him about Frank. So Errol having lined up another date, promptly rang back to ask if my friend and I would like to join him and Molly at a dance in Booborowie. We accepted and went in Errol's car. He was the only man of my acquaintance who owned a brand-new car and we all enjoyed the night.

The next time he asked me out was some months later in November when visiting Ivor (his father had previously died). It was a week before his departure for Canada, via England, and as I had no boyfriend, I accepted.

Frank had been transferred to Balaclava in the lower mid-north, and after eighteen months that brought an end to our relationship. Despite his apparent devotion to me, he was evidently engaged all along to a girl in Wangaratta. This was reported to Helen by a girl I knew at

Woodlands and who was now nursing with Helen. She was a cousin of Frank's and on hearing of our friendship passed on the news. As Frank had not been away from the town, except for two weeks annual holiday to his parents in Launceston, it was very hard to believe that he could be engaged to someone else, so we presumed it was broken-off or that his cousin was misinformed. Early in our friendship, I had seen studio photographs of two girls in his room, and when questioned he had said one was his sister and the other his sister's best friend! No doubt, she was his fiancée.

I still find it difficult to believe that anyone could accept our hospitality, and deceive both my parents and me over eighteen months - not to mention being so disloyal to his fiancé. Whether he was trying to decide between the two of us, I will never know. English novels would describe him as a cad. Sometime later Helen passed on that he had indeed married his fiancée!

In October 1951, Paul visited Burra for a couple of days on his way to Broken Hill. He had quite a lucrative business buying second-hand cars in Melbourne, doing them up and selling at a profit wherever he could. While in Burra, he stayed at the Burra Hotel and helped Dad to construct a 'do-it-yourself' kit garage in our driveway. He asked if I would like to go to Broken Hill with him. As my mother had grown up in that city and I had not been there, I was very keen. Unexpectedly, Mum and Dad agreed to my going. Doubtless Paul had ingratiated himself to Dad by his assistance with the garage, and besides he had a persuasive and very likeable personality. We drove up to Broken Hill and to my surprise on our arrival at the hotel, Paul booked us in to separate rooms. There were several possible reasons for this: the receptionist might ask for proof of marriage, as a precaution in case my parents checked in an emergency, or that he had been there before with someone else, which was the thought that came first to my mind!

Paul had another passion besides girls and cars, which was horseracing, developed over years as an only child going to races in Melbourne with his parents. I rather fancy that betting on the horses was quite profitable for him. So, on Saturday afternoon we went to the

Broken Hill races, a memorable and colourful event exactly as portrayed by the artist Pro Hart in many paintings. Whether the reason for visiting Broken Hill was to attend the races or to sell the car, and whether or not the car was actually sold, I do not know. I returned home by the Adelaide express and Paul went back to Melbourne. On the train I met two boys, who on learning that I came from Burra asked about forthcoming dances in the town. I told them about a ball coming up in the following weeks and they immediately expressed interest, asking if they came would I accompany them, to which I agreed.

The ball coincided with Errol's next visit to Burra. His first invitation was to the high school where Ivor and others were playing table tennis. I was not into table tennis and told him so, but he insisted that it was of no importance so I went. I remember sitting on the stage watching the players, while he dazzled me with figures and talked about the wonders of the newly acquired room-size computer installed in the offices of the smelters at Port Pirie where he worked. I did not understand half of what he said but that seemed to go unnoticed, and did not deter him from asking me to drive to Clare for lunch the following day. As it was Saturday, this presented a slight problem. I had by then returned to working in the bank, which was open until 11:30 on Saturdays, and no one could leave until all staff had balanced the books. I recall seeing Errol walking up and down outside in the street patiently waiting for me to emerge (he would say he has been waiting for me ever since). It was a romantic drive over to Clare and our first lunch was celebrated in a fish cafe, which was the only place open but still romantic.

Only once before had I been out to dinner with a young man. Mervyn Longford, a grazier who lived a distance from Burra, was very keen on me for years. He was about eight years older and although he was very nice, I considered that he was too old for me. We went together to many dances and to the pictures. I recall the occasion he took me to dinner at the Kooringa Hotel where we had a bottle of sauterne (my first taste).

A Quality Life

After I left Burra to go overseas he married a girl younger still, who obviously did not think he was too old. Almost fifty years later at the Back to School, I met Mervyn and his wife Shirley with whom I had played tennis. I made some flippant remark to him about our past: he looked at me blankly as though he had no idea who I was. Indeed! He had pursued me intently! Once when meeting him on the train to Adelaide, he asked where I would be staying. I replied that I would be with my Auntie Nora and he pressed me for the address, which I gave him. The following day I received a phone call from him, asking me to go out. In order to obtain the telephone number, he had gone through the entire directory checking the address I had given him. He had no idea that Auntie Nora's surname was Wincey being right at the end of the directory. A sign of true and devoted love, I thought, and yet he had so easily forgotten me! I was quite thrown by his non-recognition, and decided that being over seventy he must be suffering from dementia!

The Saturday after our lunch at Clare was the night of the ball, and despite Errol's protests, I insisted that the two young men from Adelaide pick me up and take me as I had promised them. Errol made it quite clear however, that once there he would not leave me alone. Later when dancing with me he confessed that he had stood on the balcony above, while watching me dance with one of them, and had contemplated the consequences of toppling one of the huge flower-filled urns over the railing onto my partner.

Fortunately it did not come to that, as the boys got the message and were more than happy to turn their attentions elsewhere.

The ball was a great success. I was wearing my long blue velvet frock, which I had worn as Bunny's bridesmaid, and a funny badminton hat with shuttlecocks and other paraphernalia that won the most original hat prize. Errol was looking very handsome in his dark suit (dinner suits were not generally worn, though Masons always wore them to their Lodge meetings) and he escorted me home. What more could a girl want? In 1951 or in any year?

After The War

The night before his departure on the Oronsay for England, we spent the evening baby-sitting the Burdon children as Ivor and Blanche were going out. It was a wonderful opportunity to be alone on our last night together, when we discussed the future and what it might hold for us. As it so happened I had already booked my passage to England on another P&O liner, the Otranto, departing the following June 1952 shortly before my 26th birthday. Although Errol years later loved to tell people that I had followed him to England and later to Canada (the latter was true, but at his request), my passage had been booked months before any relationship with Errol started. As I also would be in the northern hemisphere and closer to Canada, this opened up the possibility of us meeting again in the not too distant future. Errol confessed he had finally met the girl with whom he would like to spend the rest of his life. It was ironic that he was on the brink of departing for the other side of the world, perhaps for years. I felt much the same way and we decided to correspond. Letter was the only practical way available to us for keeping in touch in those days. In retrospect, I realise that for us it was the best way, since one can express one's feelings so much better in the written word than in the spoken. It was a courtship maintained by letter for twenty months before we met again.

On this, our last night together, the peaceful quiet was suddenly broken by the sound of a loud horn and a knock on the front door. Errol went to the door and returned with a huge oblong box that he presented to me. I opened it revealing a literal garden of flowers, bunches of every imaginable type of flower: irises, daffodils, poppies, roses, lilies, frangipani, freesias, violets, the rare sweetly perfumed Australian native boronia and exotic orchids to mention just a few. There being no florist in Burra, Errol had ordered the flowers from an Adelaide florist. They had come by train and then collected and delivered by Teddy Lehmann to the door. The huge box was the type used by florists when sending flowers to churches and reception rooms in preparation for a wedding. I had never been given flowers before, nor had anyone I knew, and it was not the usual custom for young men to do so. Apart from bunches of violets, boronia and spring flowers sold at the city market, from the flower carts on city street corners and Adelaide railway station, flowers were a luxury. Most people had gardens, but not the variety of exotic blooms available from a florist, who in the main supplied flowers for weddings and funerals. When his ship docked in Fremantle, Western Australia, he arranged to send by air another bunch of boronia, as it was a native of that state. It was his farewell on leaving Australian shores and confirmed his first declaration of love. Now after almost fifty years of our marriage, the true romantic that he is, he has not let a week pass without his coming home with flowers. Not quite so romantic was his attempt to seduce me in 1951 when sitting in his car. Our passions were aroused and he obviously desired 'to have his way' with me. He asked me to reach into his pocket and to my amazement, I drew out a ten-shilling note, leading me to the obvious conclusion that I was to be paid for the favour! Excuses and apologies followed, and then the final explanation that he had directed me to the wrong pocket - not the one containing the condom! Seeing the mislaid condom, I did accept his explanation, but in the confusion the moment was lost.

In between resigning from the bank the first time, when employees returned from the war and took up their old jobs, and when I re-joined in early 1951, I was a lady of leisure. Darling old-fashioned Dad insisted there was no need for me to work. Mum had not been too well and I could help her at home. I enjoyed this time, a period of around eighteen months when I took up golf, playing with the married ladies midweek and mixed at the weekends. It was only a nine-hole course and a pretty rough one at that. Fairways were just grass and ground 'au naturel', certainly not mown but perhaps stones were removed, and the 'greens' were slag from the mine. There was a huge slagheap on the hill behind the school, and beside the route taken by children from Burra North. This slag was residue from days bygone, when ore was smelted in the huge chimney that stood majestically beside it. The golf course was hazardous, providing plenty of challenges. I also took up contract bridge (auction was rarely played), and in the evenings played with three friends at either Mary Rowe's home above The National Bank where her father was the manager, or at our house. The other players were Rae Blesing and another teacher from the high school. Mrs Rowe or Mum taught us, and served us sumptuous suppers. As I had no boyfriend in sight, I gave serious thought to my ever-present dream of travel. Auntie Kath had had two trips around the world, and another to visit Auntie Jess who was then living in England. She had thrilled me with her experiences as had Auntie Jess in her letters home. So when Mr Archer, the bank manager, asked would I consider returning to my old job I jumped at the opportunity to earn enough money to enable me to fulfil this dream. This was much to Dad's disappointment, as he wanted me to stay at home, and wait for the man who would marry me! There was little chance of this in Burra as few single men came to the town and the locals were mostly married. Anyway, I wanted to see the world and did not care whether I was married or not. Besides, a girl not married by twenty-four was already regarded a spinster, and at fault regardless of the fact that she may have turned down a dozen proposals. Consequently, many girls married anyone rather than be 'left on the shelf '. The following illustrates this. When I was about twenty-three, after my relationship with Frank was over, Helen and I had lunch in Adelaide with a former Burra boy Jim Terry, a friend of my former boyfriend Don Christie. Jim had transferred to the Sydney branch of the National Bank and had taken me out when I visited Sydney with Mum. During lunch when talking about our friends in Burra, Jim commented that as we were the only ones left in the old gang that we should get together. Helen remarked that Jim was quite serious and I should consider his proposal. I explained to her that although I liked Jim, who was very good looking and had very good job prospects, I did not like him sufficiently to take up his offer. Most unmarried girls at that time would have jumped at the opportunity, which may have turned out very well - who knows? As we are now living in Sydney, I wonder if Jim might also be here.

The whole of 1951 was devoted to saving enough money to finance my travel plans. Fortunately, bank salaries had increased considerably so it was not difficult to save. In fact, my twelve pounds a week was the same as the manager had received just a few years before, and was also more than Rae Blesing earned as a teacher. At that time and unlike today, teachers were well paid compared to other professions. It was with some difficulty I persuaded Rae to accompany me. She would have to resign from a stable position which might jeopardise her future, and as both parents were dead they could offer no financial support if she fell on hard times. She was loath to take such a step. Ultimately, she did however, and forever gave me thanks as she went on to bigger and better things.

I can now tell of an incident in 1952, not long before embarking for England. To me it was amusing though the family were very concerned for me, which I did regret. A neighbour invited me to visit him for the evening, as he needed some company. His young wife was dying of cancer and in an Adelaide hospital, so naturally he was depressed and lonely. I did not know him well since he and his wife were new to the town, so I told a white lie by leading Mum to believe that there were other people going. The evening started off harmlessly with our sitting chatting, sipping sherry, liqueur and possibly beer. In hindsight, it was quite a mixture and little wonder that suddenly I felt quite ill so went to the bathroom where I vomited. The last thing I remembered was falling down and then woke to find myself on a bed. To my horror, the time was 7 am. How would I explain my overnight absence to my parents, and worse, how to leave a married man's home at that early hour without being seen by the neighbours? The only solution was to climb over the dividing fence between our two properties and sneak into our house, into my bed, and to hope that I had not been missed. After successfully avoiding Dad in the kitchen, the subterfuge really took off from there. At the time, Fuff was staying with us and I had almost reached my bedroom when I heard her call out to Mum, 'She's not in bed.' As she moved away, I was able to sneak undetected into my bed. The deception took off in mammoth proportions when I heard Mum phoning Dad who had since gone to work. A very worried Dad promptly went across the road to Elder Smiths, where my host worked, to inquire whether I had left his house safely and soundly the previous night. On hearing that I had, Dad reported back home so Fuff checked my bed again and lo and behold, there was June snug as a bug in a rug! To my shame, I vehemently denied Fuff's assertion that I had not been in bed earlier, claiming that I had been there all night long. Fuff was unconvinced but puzzled, I think, as to how I managed to get into bed between her checking twice, though I believe that the first time she just looked in from the doorway. I dared not tell her the truth as she would surely have told Mum and Dad (I wouldn't have blamed her). Although I was aged twenty-four, it would have led to all sorts of explanations. I hope that she forgives me and finds it amusing when she reads this.

To venture abroad

Rae Blesing and I booked our passage on the one-class ship SS Otranto, leaving Adelaide for Southampton, June 1952, shortly before my twenty-sixth birthday. I spent a whole year planning the trip. I bought a huge second-hand leather trunk, which was advertised in The Advertiser, and two new matching suitcases, one large and one small. I mended all my underwear as we threw out nothing unless ragged. I organised my vast wardrobe and things I might need, even including my tennis racquet, golf clubs (all four of them!) and golf bag, with the view to including Canada in my itinerary. How different and easier it is today, with the young setting out for the unknown with a backpack (often packed the night before), as all our three children have done. I still have the trunk and suitcases, which are now filled with mementos and special clothes.

All preparations, however, added to the excitement as I packed. Of utmost importance was obtaining a passport (British) from Canberra. Despite all the talk and activity in our household, when my passport arrived by post, dear Dad asked what was it for. He preferred to believe that I was not going. On the boat before our departure, he said quietly to Rae that he expected he would not see me again, which shocked me when Rae told me later. Strangely, it was my mother who would miss me most, as I was the only daughter living at home we spent so much time together ... yet she gave me every encouragement. She had always wanted to travel like her sisters, Kath and Jess, and so understood. Besides, she knew about my feelings for Errol and my hopes of meeting him in Canada. She had been as excited as I was, when six months earlier I had returned home laden with flowers, which filled every vase and room in the house.

The day arrived for our embarking on the Otranto. Dad drove Mum and me to Adelaide for its departure. The previous day there had been heavy rain flooding vast areas in the Lower North. As we approached Adelaide, one road was knee-deep in water, and even with the very high chassis and mudguards, it was impossible to attempt to drive the car through safely. Fortunately, there was sufficient time for us to turn back and try a different route. Eventually we arrived at Outer Harbour where all the liners normally berthed. Many of our close relatives and friends were there to farewell us. All the passengers and their guests went on board to inspect the cabins and what was to be our home for the next four weeks.

Fuff, Helen and Guy met us at the dock. (Peg by then was living in Brisbane.) Guy was attending Scotch College in Adelaide as a boarder, since Mum was very keen for Guy to have a private school education such as her three brothers had received.

On the ship, my cousin Deidre introduced me to a friend who had been an airhostess with her at TAA (Trans Australian Airlines, now part of Qantas). Marika and her friend Doff (Dorothy) Savage were also sailing. They were both from Kempsey, NSW and we all became good friends while aboard. Since then, we have all kept in touch at Christmas. Years later, when I was living in Tasmania, Doff wrote to say she, her husband and their small children were moving from near Kempsey to Hobart. Though both living in Tasmania, only three hundred kilometres apart, we never managed to meet until after I had moved to Sydney. Doff and I eventually met again after thirty years, when I went to Hobart for Jennifer's university graduation. Jennifer knew one of Doff's sons, Bill, who was also graduating and unbeknownst to me they had organised our meeting. Many times since, I have met Doff while in Hobart visiting Jennifer.

Also on board the ship was a special friend Jeanette Thomas from Broken Hill. She later married an Englishman Peter McHenry and several years on returned to Adelaide to live and raise five children. We all maintained a close friendship until Jeanette's death late last year in December 2001.

The Otranto was the first one-class liner and was on her second voyage from Australia to the United Kingdom. Travelling one-class was very popular for the many single girls setting off for Europe, and consequently the majority of my generation fell into that category. Apparently, Ruth Cracknell, the well-known actress, was on our voyage though I do not recall her. I have since discovered that Gwen Cordner, a Sydney friend, was on the first voyage that departed in February of 1952.

Few young men could risk their future by leaving their steady jobs. Mostly they were still the breadwinners and their jobs were for life. Errol had a friend, who had moved to Canada, and reported that as an accountant he would have no difficulty finding work, which proved to be the case. In Canada, men frequently changed jobs to advance their careers, though at that time men in Australia did not. As both Canada and Australia were part of the British Empire, an Australian could enter Canada as an immigrant, which was merely a matter of signing a form and having a certain small sum of money. From Canada it was simple to cross the border to the USA, though one was not allowed to work or to stay an unlimited amount of time.

What a momentous and colourful occasion it was as we steamed from the harbour to the tune of The Maori Farewell, tearfully sung by passengers and those on the wharf to the accompaniment of a band. We threw coloured streamers to the wharf where family and friends anxiously grabbed them, and we all held on tightly to our last link with each other - until the streamers eventually broke and the liner pulled away.

We steamed south down St Vincent's Gulf to The Southern Ocean, then west across the Great Australian Bight, that notoriously rough stretch of water spanning the southern coast of South Australian and Western Australia. Most of the passengers suffered severe seasickness in the Bight and spent the time in their bunks or hanging over the side of the ship. We reached Fremantle, four days after leaving Adelaide. I was one of the few who gained my sea legs quickly but had little company on deck.

Rae and I, and our new friends, had not visited Perth before and took advantage of a tour of the beautiful beaches, Perth surrounds, the university and the unique shopping mall - Tudor Court. Perth like all Australian cities is much changed now, and Fremantle has since had a complete makeover reflecting its colourful past. It is a fascinating place to visit, whereas in 1952 it was a very drab port.

Our two-berth cabin was small but quite adequate for two single girls, and I would not have cared to be in a four-berth, least of all in a six. We had a dressing table between our bunks and a wardrobe. After unpacking necessities and some clothes, our cases were removed to the hold where we could go at certain hours each day to collect any clothes we might need; especially for dinner as we always dressed up at night. My trunk, which had been sent by train direct to the ship, was also in the hold together with others. It was not required for the voyage as it held clothes for future use in England and possibly Canada. The laundry and ironing rooms were nearby and we made good use of those facilities, as all frocks required ironing. Fortunately, the toilet and bathroom were also very close to our cabin.

Life on the high seas

The next few weeks more than fulfilled any expectations. Although it was a one-class ship, it was a luxurious experience without the snobbery often associated with first-class travel. Despite this last comment, Auntie Kath had reported that on her last trip returning first-class to Australia, her fellow passengers included Italian migrants, who had no respect for the fine appointments of the lounges and dining room, shown by a habit of wiping their mouths on the tablecloths. After the war when many migrants paid ten pounds to come to this country, they were often filled with such people, and as a consequence, many ships required much refurbishment afterwards.

I believe we each paid one hundred and thirty pounds Australian for our two-berth cabin, about thirty pounds more than the cost per person for a four berth. We felt the difference was well worth it and very reasonable. This fare covered everything on board (entertainment, food, wine served with meals), in fact everything except for drinks from the bar. Errol's first class ticket for a two berth (he was accompanied by a friend, Don Hastings as far as England) was a further thirty pounds on a more luxurious liner. However this added luxury had its drawbacks as there were many older couples and dowagers on board, and only a few young single girls with whom the two men could while away the romantic, moonlit tropical evenings. Our situation was the reverse regarding young males, however at least all passengers in the main were reasonably young. I also believe that in first-class it was expected that men should wear dinner suits and ladies evening dress, whereas one-class was a little more casual, jackets and ties for men, and frocks for women.

It was a true holiday in every sense. Each morning at seven, we were awakened by our Indian cabin-steward knocking on the door with tea and biscuits. Then followed two sittings of breakfast (8a.m and 9 a.m.) when we were indulged with every manner of porridge, breakfast cereal, tropical fruits, and various egg, fish, savoury hot dishes and toast. The Indian waiters were expertly trained by the British as to the fine etiquette of the table, and no one does it better than the Indians. The officers were British and the rest of the crew mostly Indian, if my memory serves me right.

Our days were occupied with swimming in the pool and playing numerous deck games: quoits, table tennis and deck tennis to name a few. The more skilled entered competitions, for which prizes were given at the end of the voyage. On his trip, sporty Errol won a few, including quoits, table tennis and greasy pole where contestants sat astride a slippery pole and endeavoured to push each other off and into the pool below. He still has one prize, a silver ashtray with the flag and name of the SS Oronsay on it. From memory, I believe that I too won something but have nothing to show for it now. In between more active pursuits, we spent a lot of time sunning ourselves, reading or just happily lazing on deck, gazing dreamily at the Indian Ocean skimming by and the ever-changing cloud formations in hazy tropical skies.

Mid-morning, waiters carried around Bovril (a beef tea drink) and dry biscuits to energise us, and mid-afternoon the ritual was tea on deck, or tea and cakes in the lounge. As with breakfast, lunch consisted of four or five courses served in the dining room. Dinner was the most formal and so pre-dinner there was much activity below deck as we ironed our frocks, showered, and prepared ourselves. Dressed in our finery, we entered the dining room where the officers lined up to welcome us before joining us at the tables. At the start of the voyage we were allotted a table at our preferred sitting, whether first or second, and throughout the voyage an officer sat at the head of each table. The waiters presented us with the menu of the day, and there were always seven courses. It was expected that we would partake of all seven, and while it seems hard to believe now, that was not a problem. We started with appetiser followed by soup, fish, entrée, main, dessert and petit fours (tiny fancy cakes). With the exception of the main, all the courses were small.

In the evenings we had a full programme of entertainment, listening or dancing to the band, games and bridge, all of which we enjoyed. Possibly films were shown but I do not recall. There were special evenings, like fancy dress, when we used all our ingenuity to conjure up costumes from materials at hand. As often happens when resources are limited people came up with many imaginative ideas.

Dinner, as with breakfast and lunch, was relaxed and lively, and spent getting to know each other, making friends and chatting about the day's activities. As we dressed for dinner and the Captain and officers attended, every evening was special to us, like going out to dinner. Each night different passengers were invited to sit at the

Captain's Table, a privilege for the selected few. After dinner we adjourned to the lounge for coffee, served black in demitasse cups with brown coffee crystals if desired. This was the time to smoke cigarettes, which most of us did. Many did so for the first time and some like me had little experience. For the next year I had an occasional cigarette, but as I did not particularly care for them, I discontinued the habit.

Highlights of the voyage were the ports of call. Approximately five days after leaving Australian shores, we reached Ceylon's port of Colombo. There was an air of great excitement as it was our first sighting of a foreign country and its people, and a way of life so different from our own. As the Otranto slowly approached the wharf, small boats came out to greet us. We had a day to enjoy this stopover and learned that the place to start was the renowned Galle Face Hotel. On the Bay of the same name, it was situated high on the hill overlooking the harbour. Immediately, we grabbed the first available rickshaw. It was pulled by a smiling Ceylonese man, who made his living ferrying around passengers from the liners. On reaching the hotel we were content to sit on the balcony, sipping cool drinks until lunch, after which we visited the very beautiful Botanical Gardens with its profusion of glorious and highly intoxicating perfumed flowers and trees in bloom. Here we were enthralled and horrified at the same time by snake charmers, who seductively played their flutes and charmed the snakes to curl around their necks and bodies. Monkeys performed and played on the ground and through the trees, showing-off their talents. We had no time to notice the intense humidity as we wandered through the markets seeking out Indian souvenirs, especially the black carved elephants as collected by every traveller to India and Ceylon in the pre-war and post-war years.

Thrilled by our first taste of a foreign culture, we happily returned to the comforts of our hotel waiting in the harbour. At sunset, we pulled away from the wharf to the sound of music and more streamers. As land disappeared from sight so did the tiny boats with the owners peddling their wares at last-minute bargain prices. Purchases and money were exchanged by means of a primitive and unique system of baskets, thrown up to the ship's deck and back again to the vendor.

At some point, we crossed the Equator and all were thrown into the pool to earn the customary certificate of proof signed by King Neptune. I do not remember the date but still have said certificate in my trunk with my other souvenirs. I did not keep a diary but now have the letters I wrote to my parents. These may be difficult to read as they were written on that flimsy blue paper of air letters.

Within the next few days we were in The Arabian Sea with the Arabian Peninsula to our north and approaching our next port of call Aden (now Al Aden - little Aden) in the Gulf of Aden. Again we had a day ashore, touring the port and nearby hinterland. Never had we seen such desolation, poverty and housing. Mud houses piled on top of each other clung to the hills, and donkeys and goats made their way through them transporting goods and people along dirt tracks.

In sharp contrast to the dry brown countryside and sombre hues of the people, the markets were colourful with rugs, baskets and fine leather, and glistening with brassware and jewellery. All were locally made and despite the irresistibly low prices, the stall and shop owners wanted to bargain; we were only too happy to oblige. In my travels since I have seen many such tourist markets duplicated all over the world, but these were unique with local items not available in boutiques in every city of the world - as souvenirs are today. Besides, it was our first exposure to such souvenirs and above all to the thrills of bargaining.

When it was time for us to embark the vendors followed, pressing us to buy at even more tempting prices, and much to our surprise and delight expecting us to offer a still lower price. Once again a flotilla of small boats followed, almost impeding our passage. Boat owners scrambled dangerously to reach the liner, wildly gesticulating, shouting and throwing us their wares in baskets - hoping for money in return.

Continuing our voyage, we entered the Red Sea and headed towards the Suez Canal. There was strife in the area due to a dispute over ownership of the Canal and even talk of its closure, in which case we would have had to turn back and complete our voyage around the Cape of Good Hope. In fact, we were one of the last ships to get through, if not the last.

Our first sighting of the canal was one of amazement. When we saw how narrow it was, we found it hard to believe that liners bigger than ours could navigate through it and that it could be deep enough. From early morning to night, we slowly manoeuvred our way through. We stopped at Port Said but were not allowed to disembark because of unrest in the region. Passengers on earlier liners had the option of disembarking and travelling overland to Alexandria, where they joined the ship again. (Six months before Errol had done this, at a cost of course). No such option for us, as the many, armed soldiers lining the shore well demonstrated.

Rae has reminded me that at Port Said, the salesmen in the boats surrounding our ship called her Queen Mary and me Mrs Simpson! No doubt these titles were conferred on all tourists.

We entered the Mediterranean, which until then had been just a romantic vision gleaned from history, fiction and popular songs, and its blueness did not disappoint us. We sailed past Crete and were excited by our first sight of Europe. Our ship went right by the magical Isle of Capri and into Napoli harbour.

It was an early morning start for our tour to the site of the Roman city of Pompeii. In 79 AD, the city was buried under volcanic ash from nearby Mt Vesuvius in one of its many eruptions. Pompeii had been excavated, exposing remains of Roman homes, bodies and animals - all now mummified stone. Fifty years on in 2002, further excavations have revealed so much more, but in 1952, it was almost beyond belief to actually view people and their existence from a period in the first century AD. Now so many ancient sites have been uncovered that one almost ceases to be amazed. We are in an age where anything is possible and although our generation gets a thrill from seeing new inventions and discoveries, I believe that, sadly, nothing may surprise or thrill the next generation. In my lifetime I have seen innumerable wonderful sights, relics and remains from the past, including the Pyramids and tombs of Egypt, mausoleums and excavated Roman cities in Turkey, the Viking remains beneath the city of York, the original Roman city of Lutetia buried under Notre Dame in Paris, Roman aqueducts in France and Spain, magnificent still perfect Roman tiled floors in Portugal, and The Great Wall of China. I have marvelled at all of them but still the memory of Pompeii remains as clear as the more recent out-of-this-world experience of viewing The Great Wall and The Terracotta Warriors in Xian, China.

Naples was a typical busy Mediterranean port, drab but interesting. I don't recall where we lunched, but I am sure it was true Neapolitan fare, in all probability local fish served by a singing waiter. We left with sadness and to the strains of Italian melodies bidding us farewell.

Back on board we took advantage of the warm summer days, sunning ourselves in swimsuits on deck and in the pool, and every day marvelling at the fact that we were actually cruising the Mediterranean. And so to Marseilles, the old southern port of France with its seedy history of gambling, drugs and murder, not unlike Shanghai and other major ports of the day. According to many novels of the nineteenth and early twentieth century, Marseilles was also an escape route for criminals who wanted to flee the country to South America, the Far East or the Pacific Islands. Even today, one is advised that it is unwise to venture into some quarters of the port.

I am reminded of our son Trevor's experience when aged twenty-four and backpacking around Europe. He planned to visit a family friend Margaret (Minns) and her second husband Warren Hayes who lived in La Ciotat just east of Marseilles. He arrived in Marseilles by train very late at night and not wanting to disturb Margaret at that hour he decided to spend the night in Marseilles. Consequently, at one a.m., he wandered around looking for accommodation, and as is typical of major city railway stations they are not located in the most desirable areas. There were drunks lying in doorways and decidedly suspicious characters in the streets, and he spent a very uneasy night in a less than respectable hotel before continuing on to La Ciotat the next morning.

We had no such dilemma on our arrival in Marseilles, for we booked a tour that took us east along the rugged coastline with beautiful views of Marseilles and surrounding country. La Ciotat, a city of high-rise units inhabited by French and retired British expatriates, is now in this area. No such city existed in 1952, only coastline where I believe we viewed an ancient fort, but my memory is hazy. However I clearly recall our lunch, which was outdoors on the terrace of a fish restaurant overlooking the sea and Marseilles. We experienced our first taste of la cuisine francaise et un pot de vin and had an opportunity to test our spoken French with the locals. Despite the fact that Rae had taught French at high school level and I had learned French at school, our Australian accents and pronunciations did nothing to enhance the language. Rae was no more successful than I was, she will forgive me I hope, in making herself understood. Both of us are much better now. Rae, after many years teaching French in England and Australia, a stint as an au pair in France, two years in Laos, many long holidays in France, and a long-standing relationship with a Frenchman, now speaks like a native; while I too, with years of study behind me and a number of trips to France, have improved my French no end.

There is something about La France that is addictive to foreigners, though it does not affect everyone. Errol and I are two of the many who have a passion for the country and its history, for provincial life with its unchanged customs, for quaint villages and friendly villagers where one truly steps back in time, for the food and wine, and the constantly changing countryside. Though some of the French city folk are rather superior to all that is foreign, they do not detract from the overall appeal.

My first step on French soil was not my last. When I returned to Marseilles forty years later, the visit was even shorter than the first time. My husband, Errol, and I landed at the airport from where we collected a hire car and immediately drove to Lambesc, a small village east of Avignon, and spent a week touring the area. We have been in the vicinity three times but never actually visited the city of Marseilles, and though we had every intention of doing so on our last visit, we were not able to fit it in.

Our last port of call was the British colony of Gibraltar. The Rock, an amazing natural monolith almost at the water's edge, seems to rise out of the water. For the British in times of conflict it provided a safe and protected gateway from the Atlantic Ocean to the entrance of the Mediterranean and beyond, and at the same time, made it extremely hazardous for the enemy in World War II to attempt to gain access by sea to Mediterranean countries. I have the idea that for security reasons we were not allowed to go ashore, and so we remained on the ship observing with much curiosity the soldiers on guard and the unloading and loading of huge crates. At nightfall when all was done we set off on the final stage of our journey, which soon saw us steaming around the south-west tip of the Iberian Peninsula to the Atlantic Ocean and in the direction of our destination, Britain.

~o~

Photo Pages I

A gallery can be viewed at A Quality Life, www.theburdons.com.

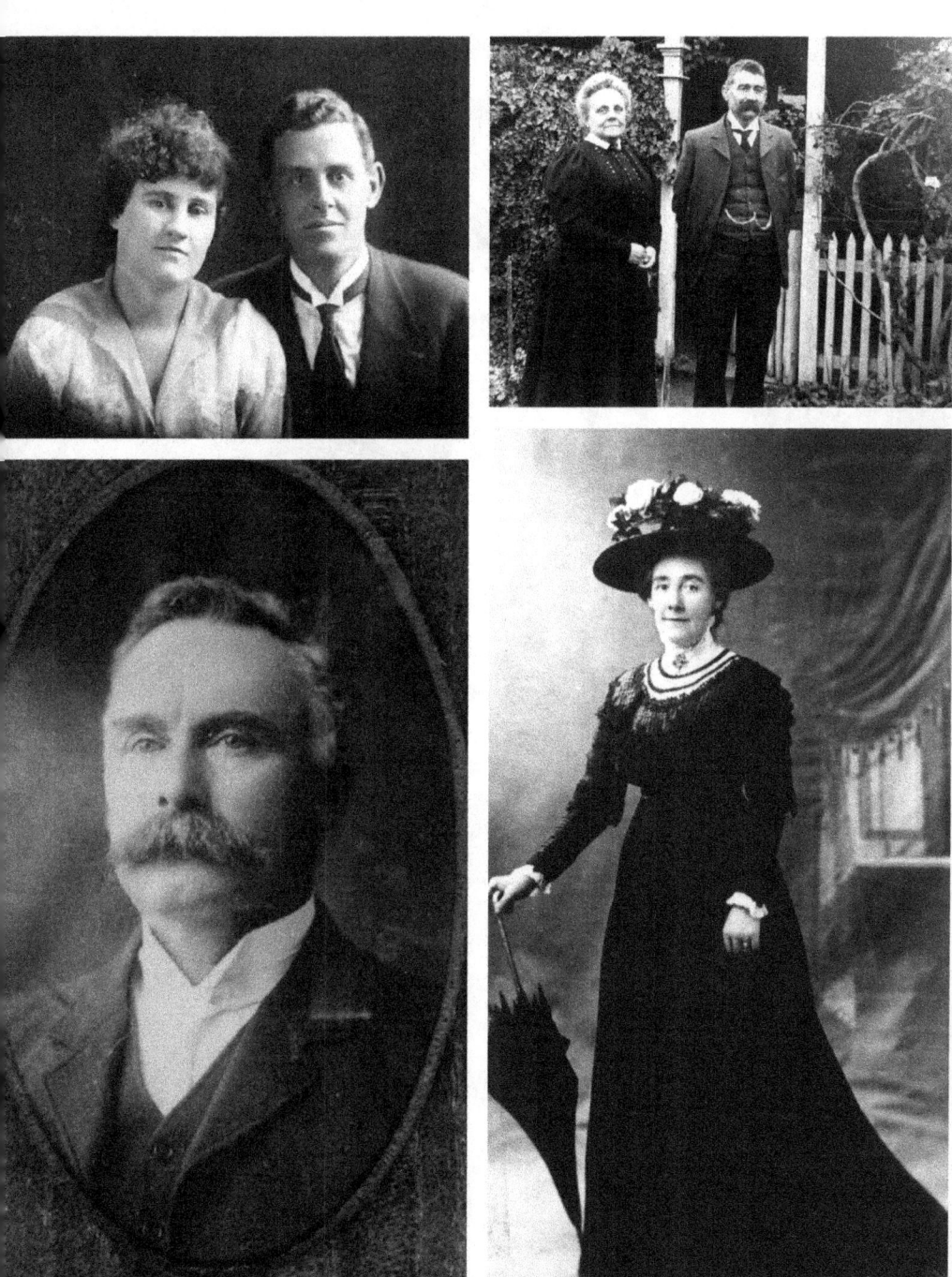

Clockwise: Parents Doris Bryant and Guy Dollman 1919; Grandparents Jane & Ernest Guy Dollman, Wilcannia 1922; Grandmother Catherine Frances Bryant 1914; Grandfather George Benjamin Bryant, Broken Hill, Christmas 1908.

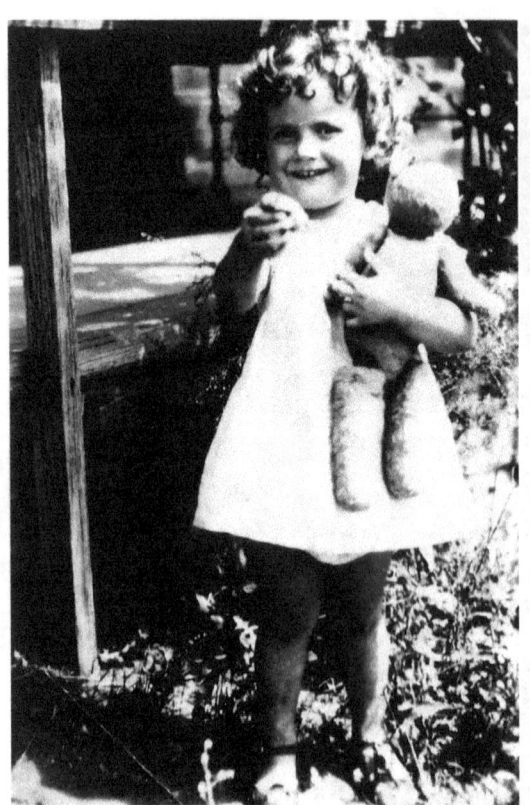
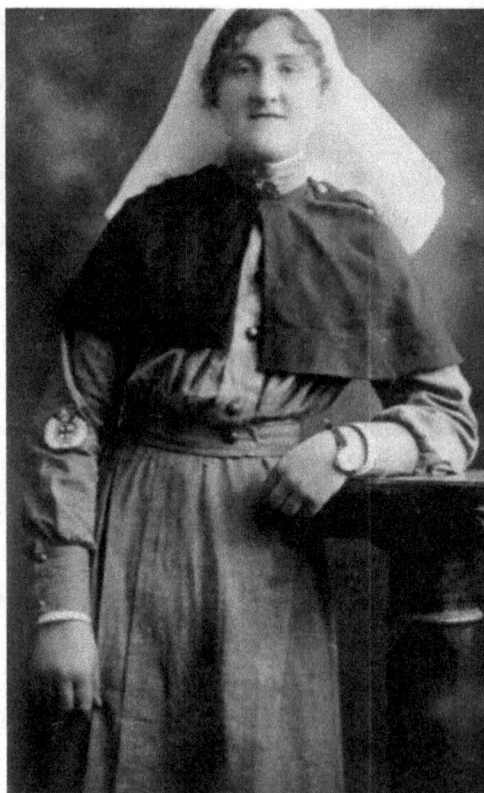
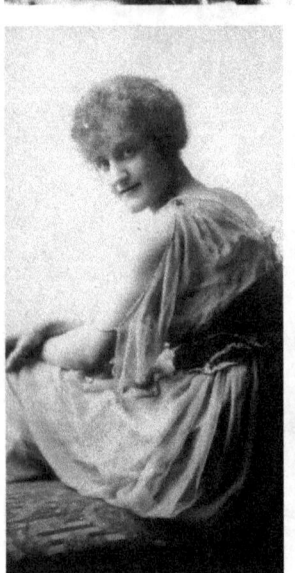
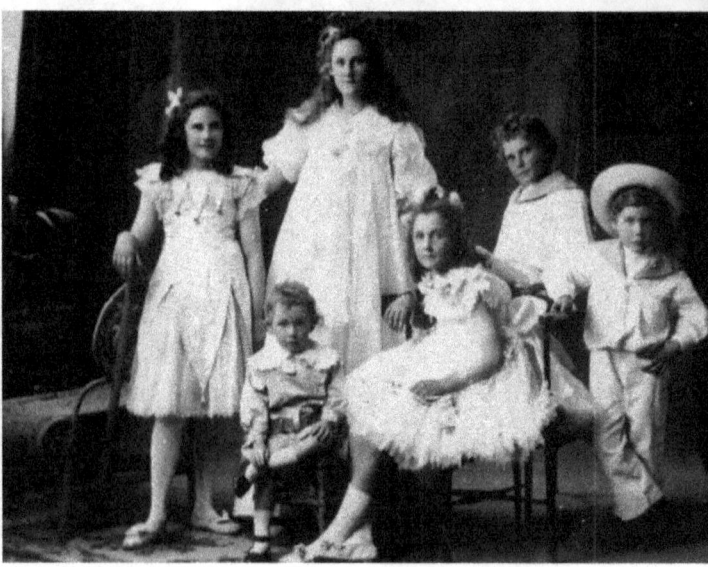

Clockwise: June with Teddy at Ware St, Burra 1928; Aunt Kath Bryant before sailing on SS Runic from Melbourne for N Africa WWI, Sep 1917; Bryant children in fancy dress, Firth, Kathleen, Jessie, Harry, Arthur, (Lenora away), Broken Hill, Christmas 1908; Aunt Jess Bryant 22 yrs. 1921.

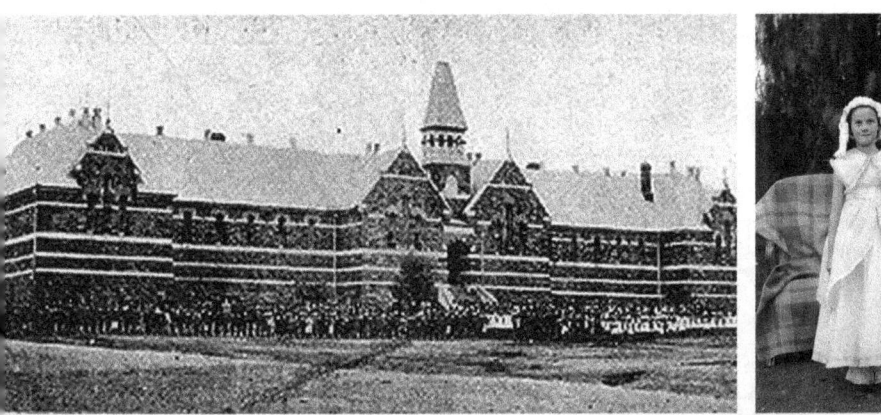
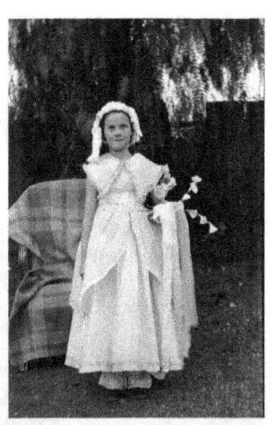
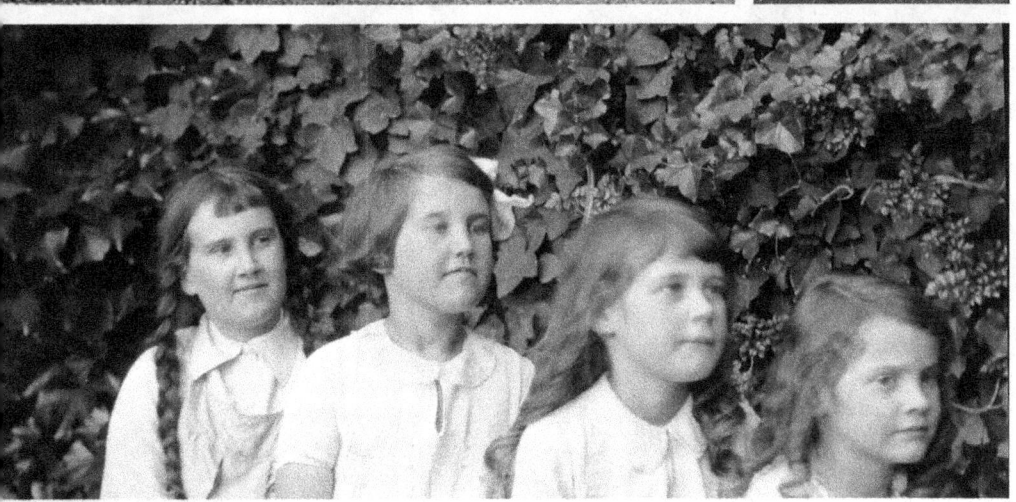
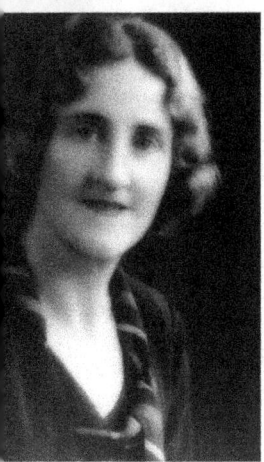
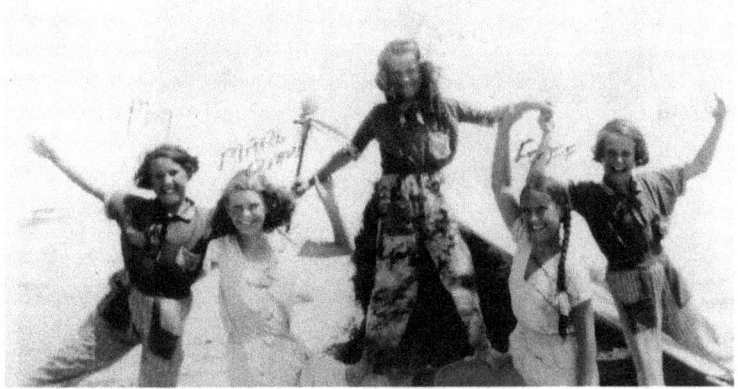

Clockwise: Burra Model School, 100th Anniversary 1936; June in fancy dress Ware St, Burra 1934 - taken by Guy H; Dolly girls Fuff, Peg, Helen & June, Hann's house Burra 1934; "Happy Dolly Holidays" - Peg,, Margaret Clark (friend), June, Fuff and Helen, Semaphore, Summer 1935/6; Aunt Kath c1925.

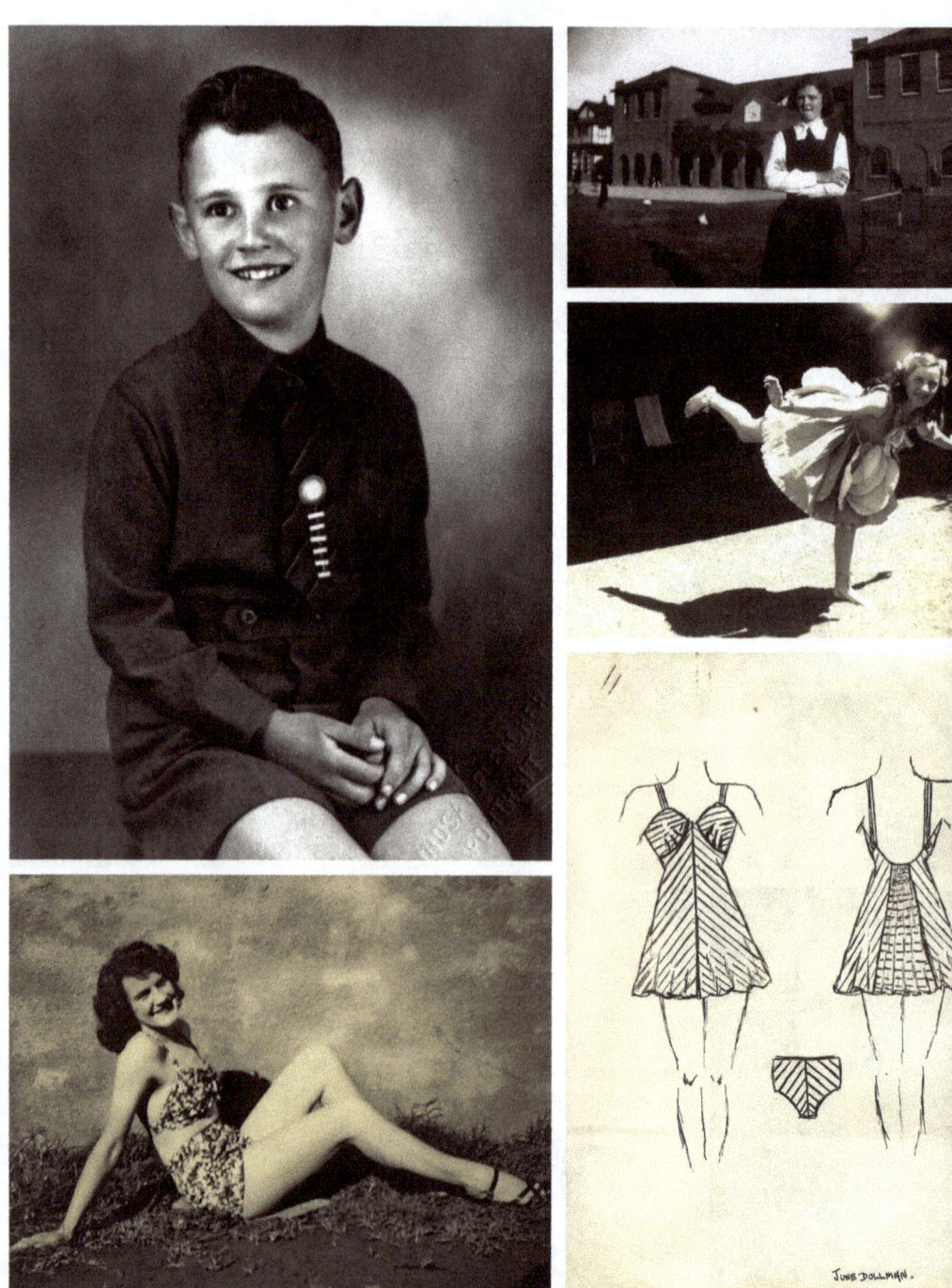

Clockwise: 'To June from Guy' Brother Guy Bryant Dollman c1946; Frizzy Fraser, Woodlands CEGGS, Glenelg c1938; June as Sweet Pea, for wartime entertainment c1942; A swimsuit competition design 1949; June modelling bathers she made, Queen St, Burra, c1946.

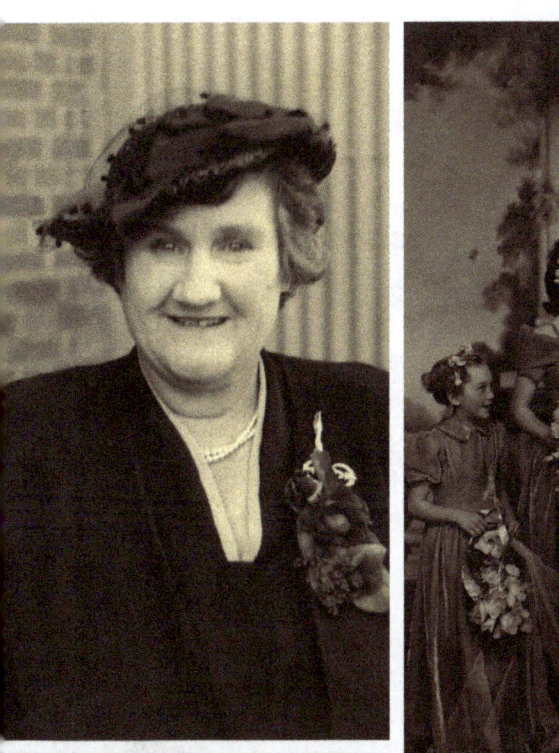
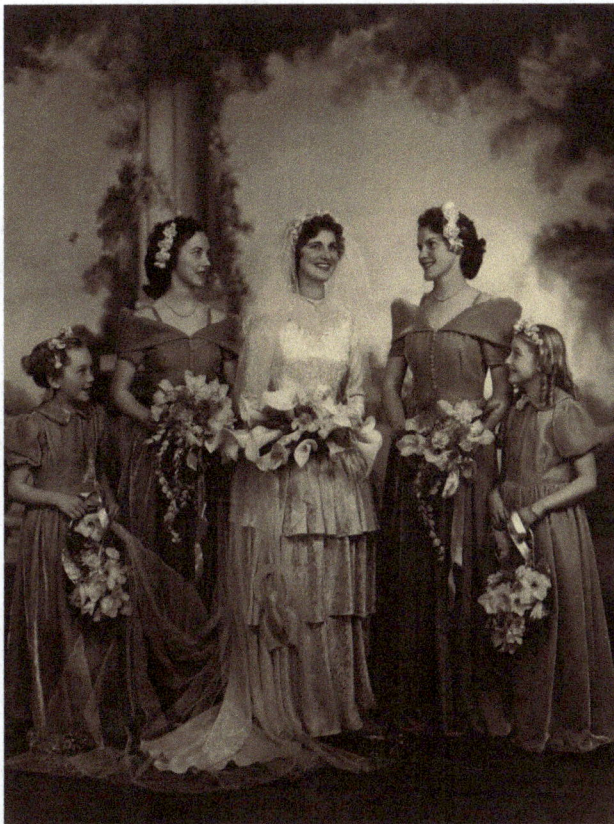
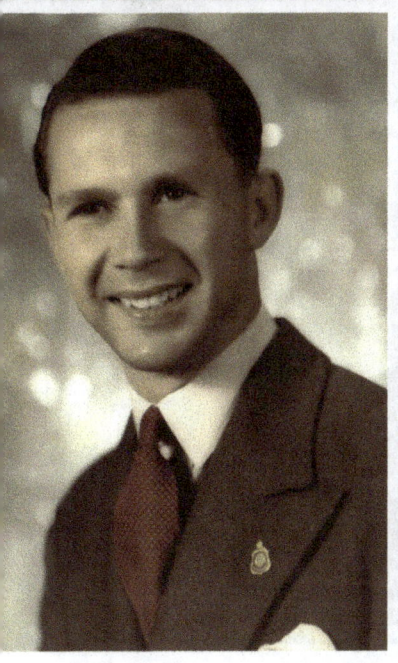
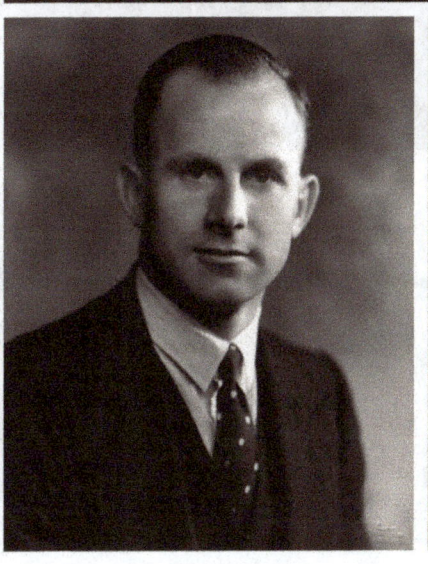
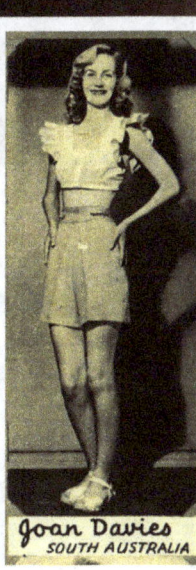

Clockwise: Mother Doris Dollman, c1951; June (right), bridesmaid to Audrey Gurney, Adelaide, 1952; Joan Davies, South Australian PIX girl Finalist, 1945; Brother-in-law to be, Ivor Burdon, 1947; Errol taken by photographer friend Clem Langsford, Port Pirie 1949 (suit by Hawkes Tailors, Adelaide).

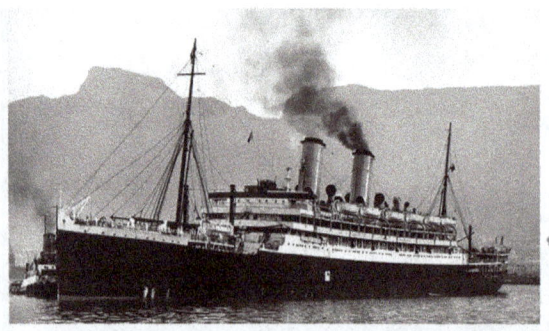
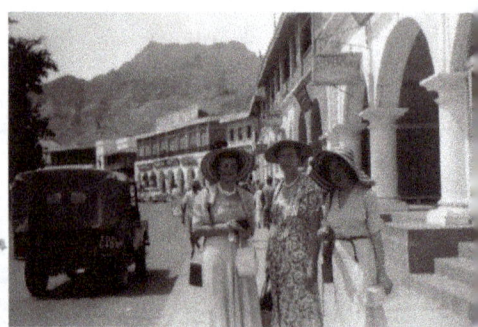
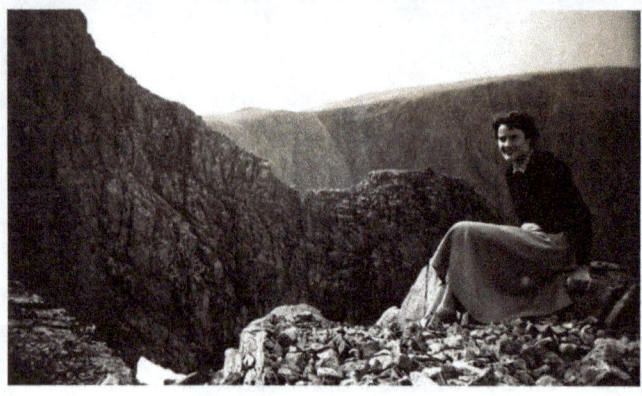
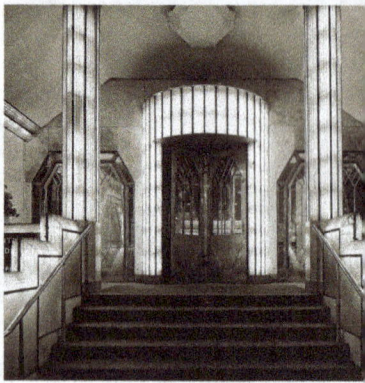

Clockwise: The single class liner, SS Otranto 1953; June, Rae & Mirella, Aden 1952; Rae Blesing & June receiving a lift from Glasgow journalists, Pass of Glencoe, Scotland, 1952; Prime lodgings. Strand Palace Hotel, London 1953; "Right on top of Ben Nevis August 1952" Scotland.

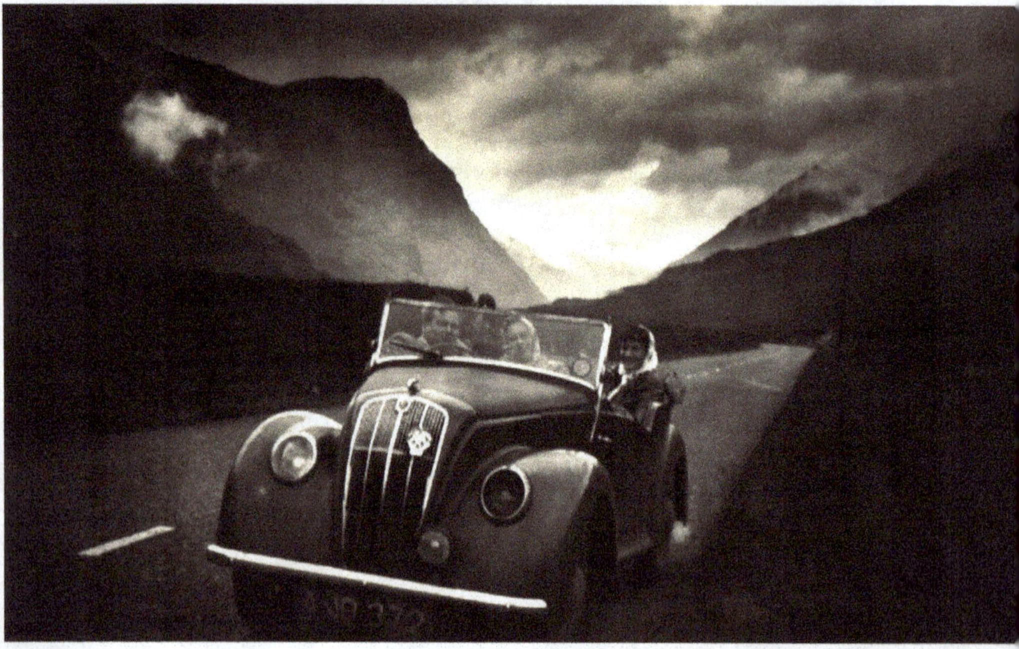

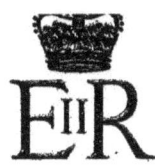

E II R

The Lord Chamberlain is commanded by Her Majesty to summon

Miss June Dollman

to an Afternoon Presentation Party at Buckingham Palace, on Thursday, the 16th July, 1953, at 3 o'clock p.m.

Ladies: Day Dress with Hats.
Gentlemen: Morning Dress or Uniform or Lounge Suit.

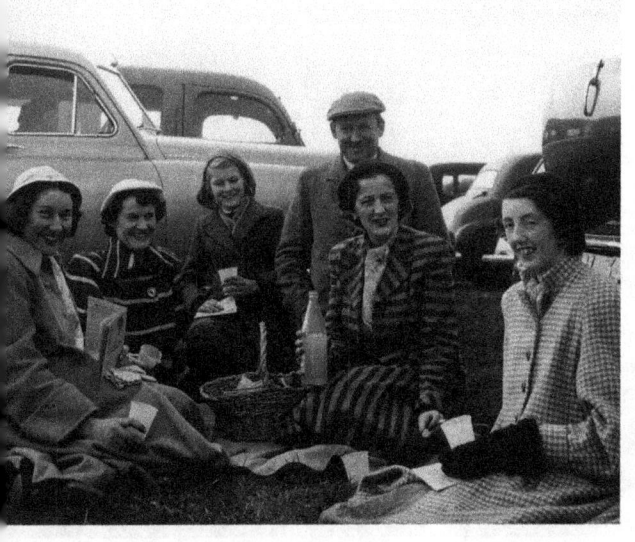
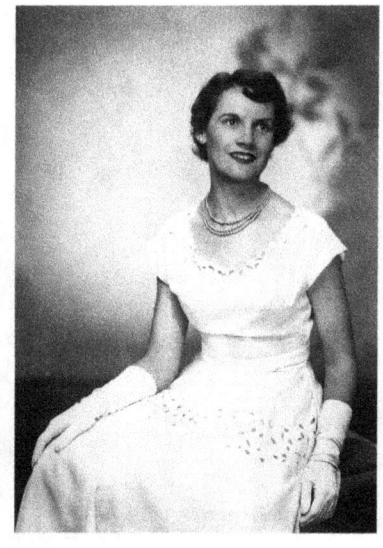

Clockwise: A Royal Command to party, Buckingham Palace, 1953; Print proof of June taken at Buckingham Palace presentation, 1953; Janette McHenry, June, Alexandra Bridgewater, Sir William & Lady Becham & Susan Jayne at Beaufort Point-to-Point Races. Taken for Tatler magazine, 1953.

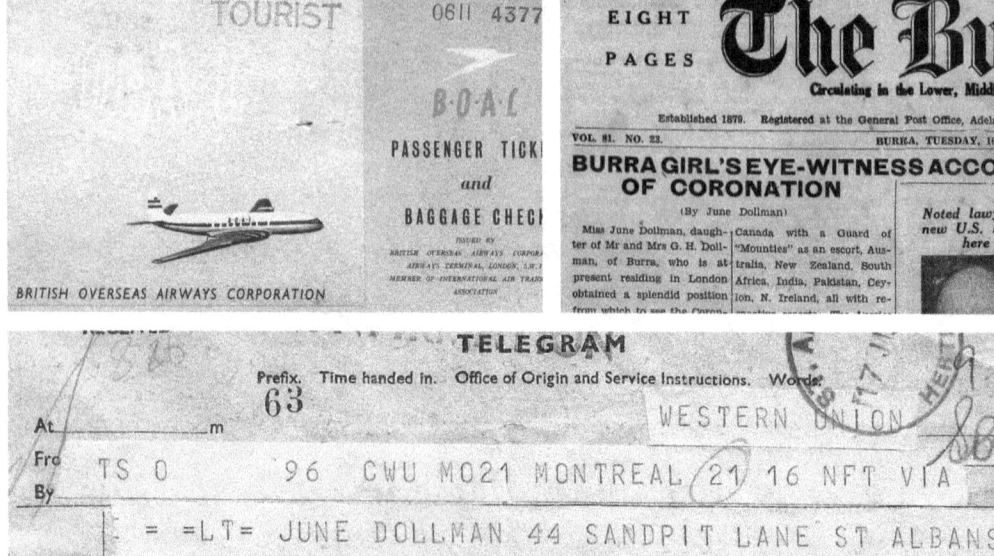

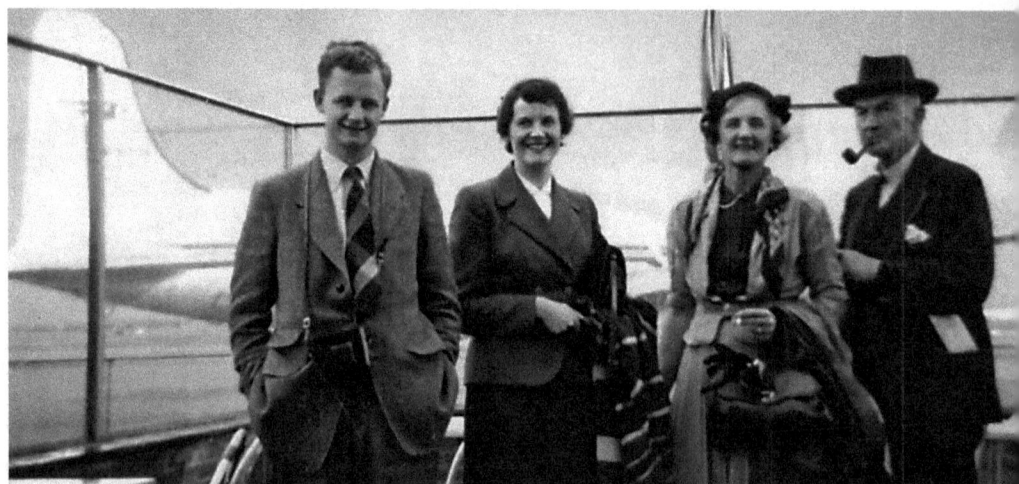

Clockwise: BOAC ticket England to Canada 1953; Roving reporter files Coronation story, Burra Record 1953; Errol's last telegram before June sets off to start a new life with him; John Miller, June, Jess Miller, Skipper Donaldson at terminal for June's flight from England to Montreal 1953.

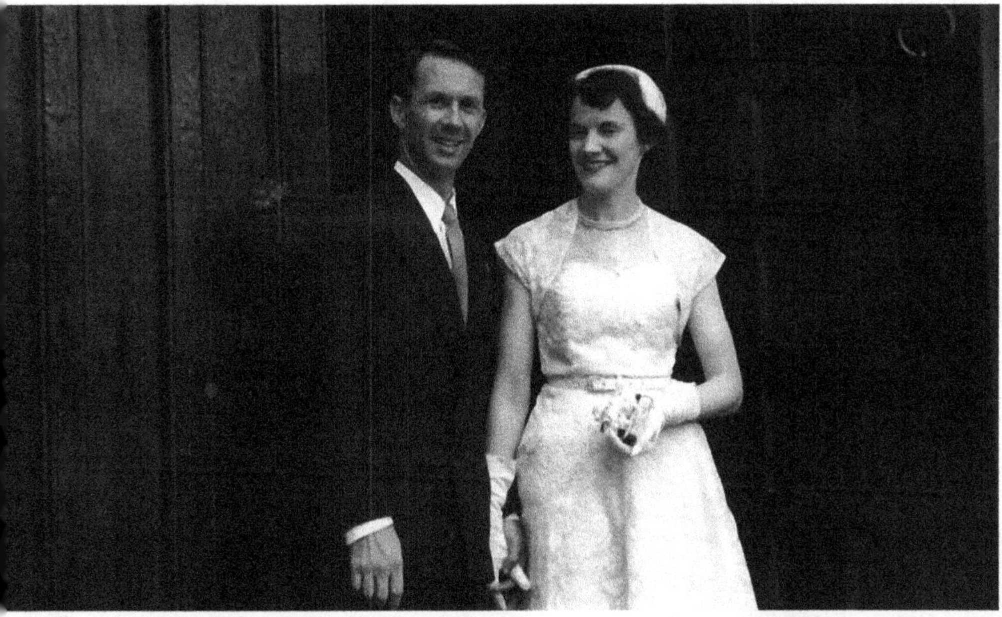

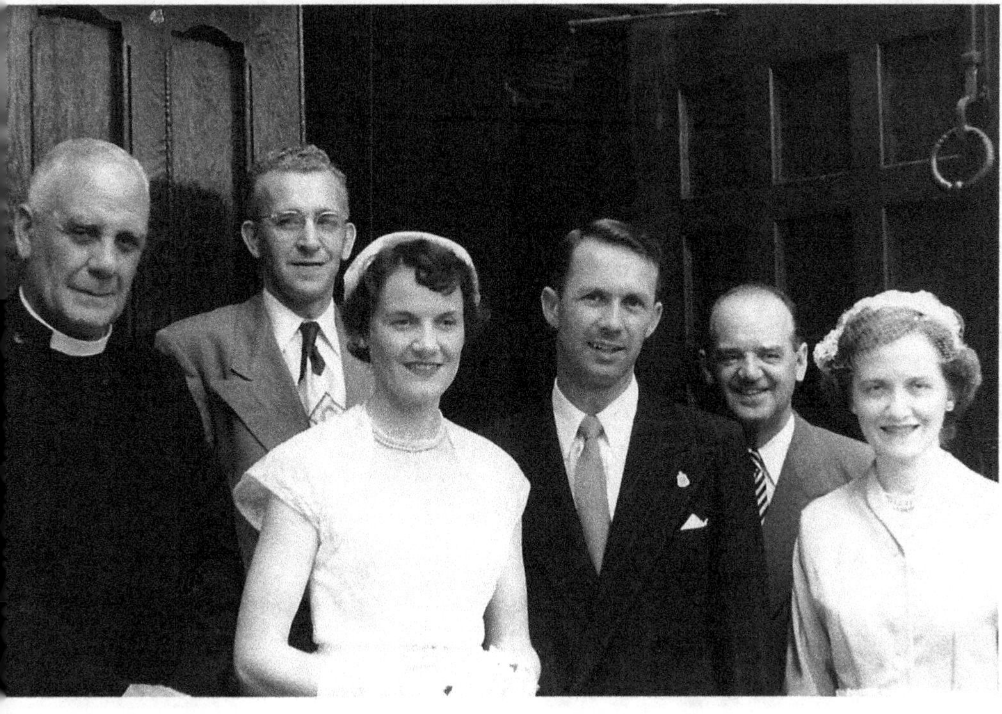

Clockwise: Wedding photo, St Mathias Church, Westmount Montreal 1953; "Rev Canon Oliver, Ed McAsey, I, Errol, Earl Younghusband, Inez McAsey. Taken by Selby McLeod 20.7.53 in front of St Mathias Church Westmount, Montreal."

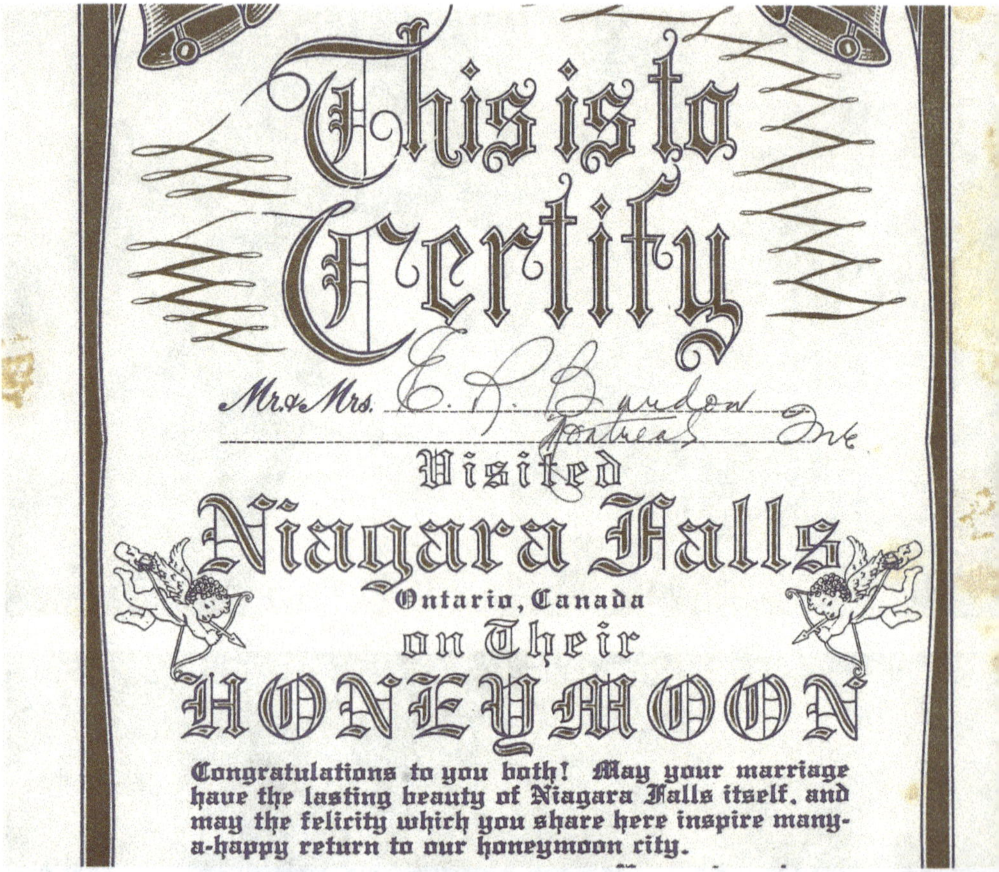

This is to Certify

Mr. & Mrs. E. R. Bardon
Montreal

Visited

Niagara Falls
Ontario, Canada
on Their
HONEYMOON

Congratulations to you both! May your marriage have the lasting beauty of Niagara Falls itself, and may the felicity which you share here inspire many-a-happy return to our honeymoon city.

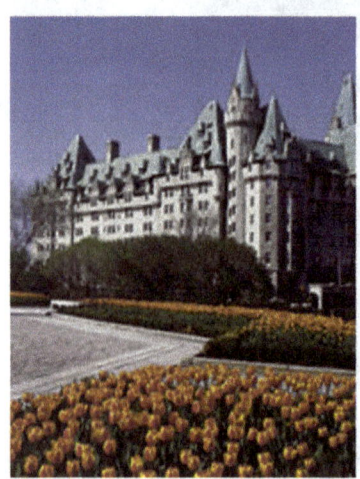

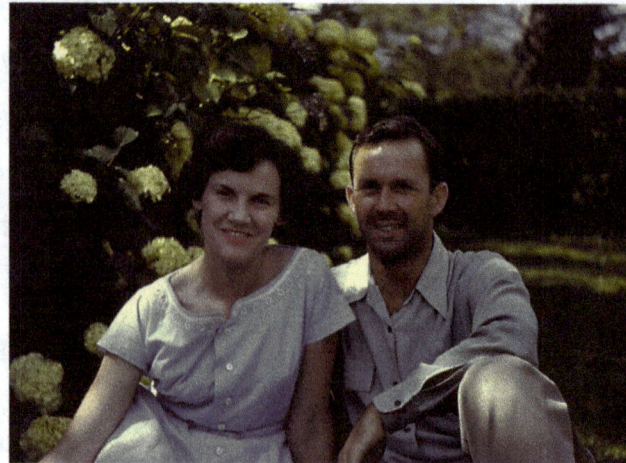

Clockwise: Niagara Falls Honeymoon Certificate, issued two years later without DOM! 1955; June & Errol Honeymoon, Ontario, July 1953; Honeymoon hotel, Chateau Laurier, Ottawa 1953.

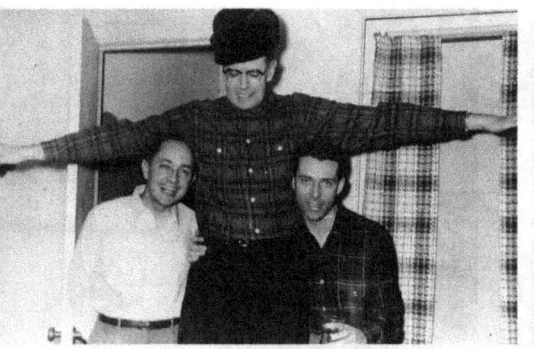
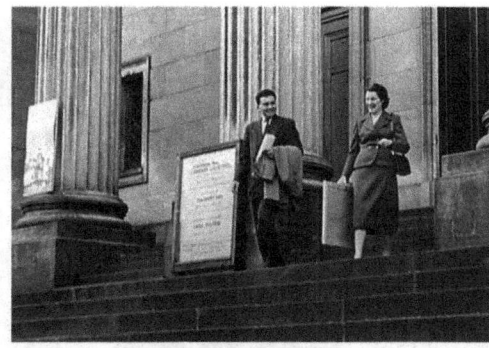
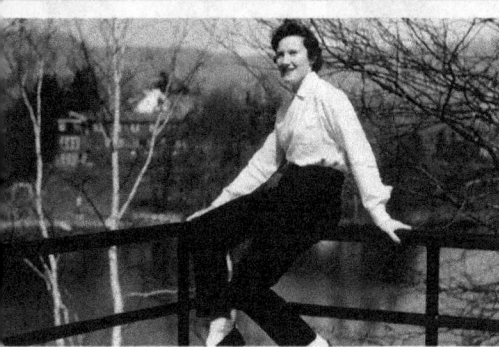
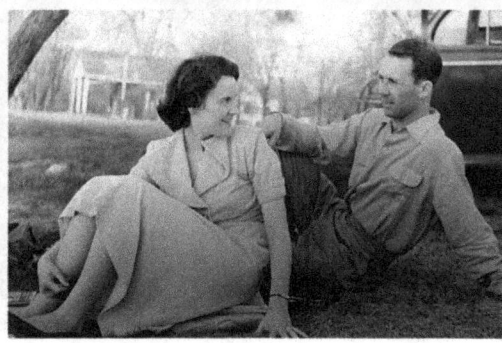

Clockwise: 1953 NYE Geoff Shannon towers over Norm Gray and Norm Bentley; "Buying or selling?" Montreal Museum, 1954; Errol & June with Mohawk guide, Appalachians, 1955; June & Errol, photo taken and developed by Errol, 1954; June lakeside at Lake Paquin with Parker Lodge in background, Laurentians, 1955.

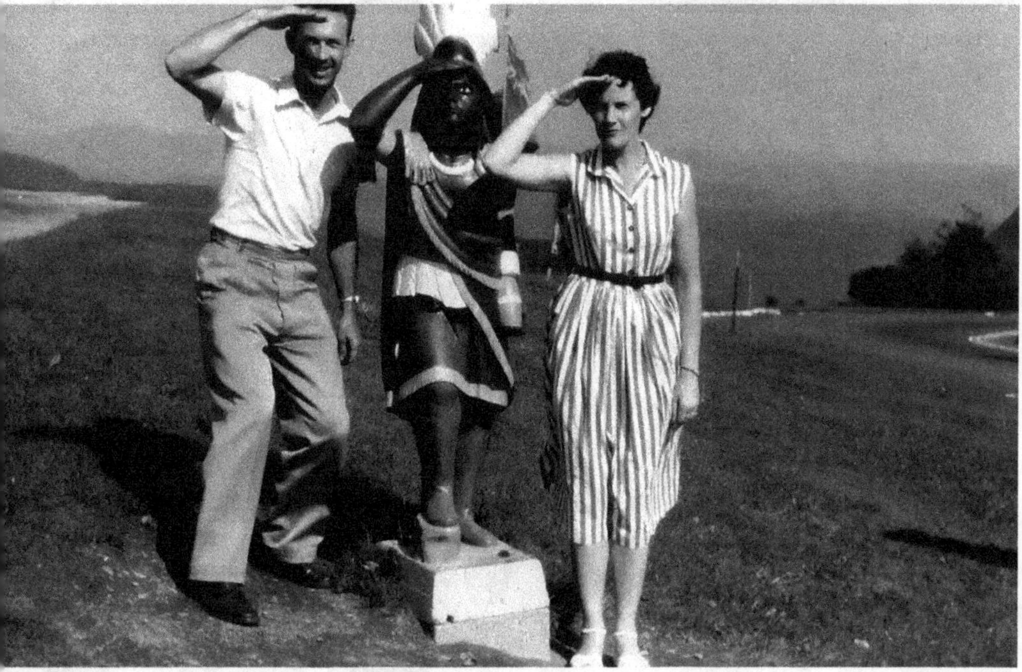

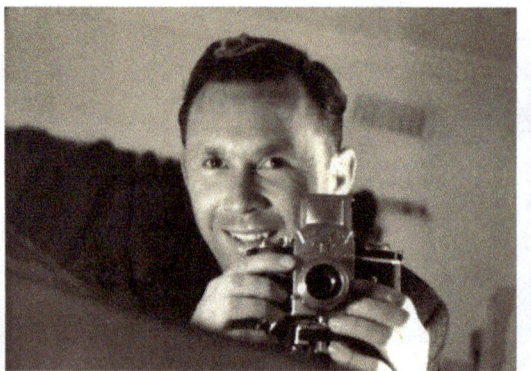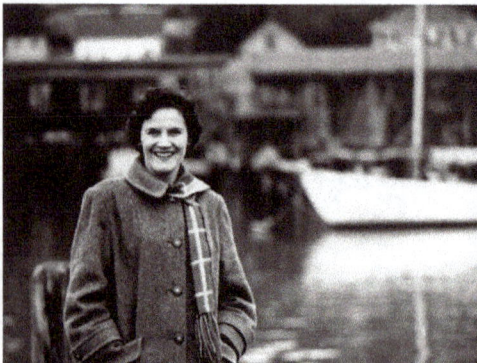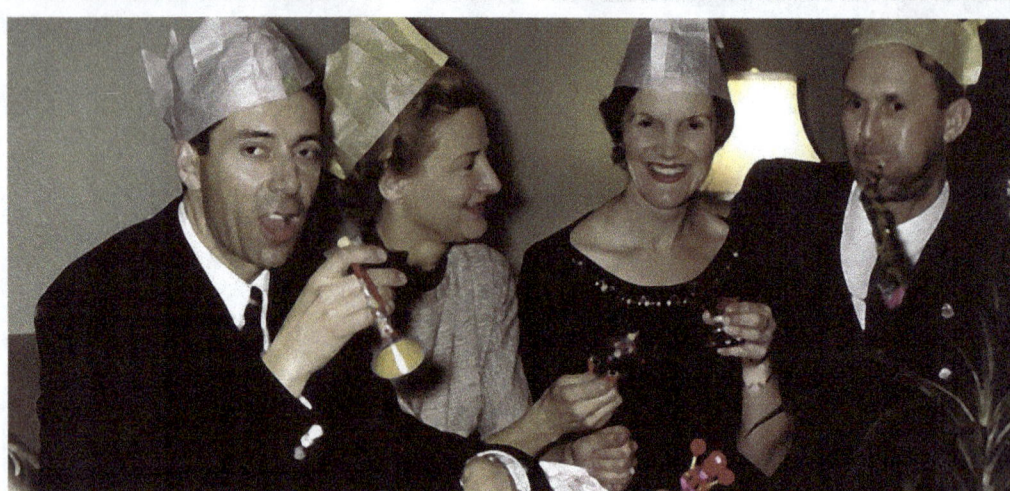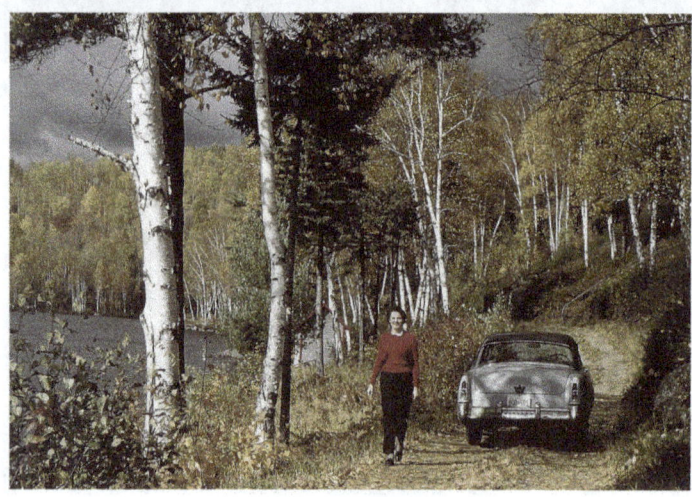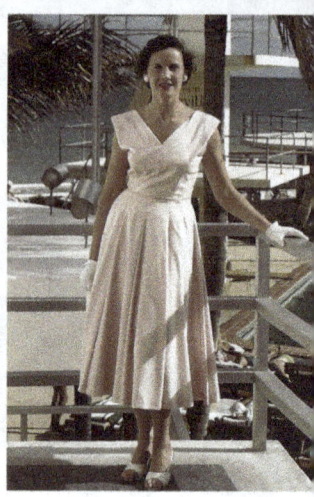

Clockwise: Errol, the man behind the camera c1955; June, Lunenburg, Nova Scotia, Sep 1957; John & Bunny Scholes, June & Errol, Montreal c1955; June poolside Hotel Seville, Miami 1955; June and Ford Monarch, Laurentian Mountains, PQ, Fall 1956.

The United Kingdom!

Within a few days, we were hurriedly packing, and exchanging addresses and promises of meeting soon with our new friends. In the midst of much sadness, tears and great excitement, we arrived at Southampton. There were more tears when I spotted Auntie Jess, who had taken the train from St Albans to London and on to Southampton, standing on the wharf. She was a favourite and special person and it was a joyful reunion after eight years apart. In no time passengers with accompanying luggage had disembarked, and were on the platform waiting for the train to London.

Arrival in London

On arrival in London Auntie Jess organised a taxi for us and our cases to the home of a widowed friend, Betty Wylie. Her husband's family were well known in Broken Hill and good friends of the Bryants. Before his death Hugh Wylie had been a Harley Street specialist (the street for all renowned London specialists of the time). Our mother had recounted the story that Hugh had failed his medical examinations several times at Adelaide University but somehow, must have finally passed and gone on to attain a PhD in England. They were the days when one paid to attend university and so many stayed on until they passed, which is starting to happen again today I believe. Betty was English and was renting out rooms in her four-storey terrace home. After we met Betty, we inspected our room and left our luggage. We rushed off to the nearby underground station for our first viewing of the more famous landmarks of London - Piccadilly Circus with all the screeching, scrambling pigeons, 10 Downing Street, Admiralty Arch, and Horse Guards Parade down the Mall with a magnificent view of Buckingham Palace; all the places we had bought and sold in our games of Monopoly and knew so well from childhood songs. We walked by St James Palace and Lancaster House, the Queen Mother's residence on Pall Mall, and then on through Green Park. At the time, it was the most thrilling moment of my life ... and it was just the start of things to come. Auntie Jess was just as excited as we were, as after eight years she never had tired of all the joys of London. After a very full and exciting day, we had a meal, then Auntie Jess returned by train to St Albans and we to our new home.

York Gate

Seven York Gate, NW1 was an exclusive address. It was so exclusive that we could never find it on any detailed map of London though the famous London cabbie who knows every inch of London like the back of his hand had no difficulty in finding it. I believe that many years later I tried to locate it on a map, again unsuccessfully. York Gate was a very short street with Regent's Park at one end and two streets away from the other end were the famed Madame Tussauds Waxworks and Marylebone Station. To reach the latter we had to cross Baker Street, made famous in the detective stories of Sir Arthur Conan Doyle as the home of Sherlock Holmes. This location being so close to the underground and just a short ride to the centre of London and its numerous attractions was ideal for us.

Rae and I had a delightful room at the back of the house on the ground floor leading into a private high-walled garden for our sole use. There was only one shared bathroom on the second floor, so much to our dismay we were allotted a set time for bathing but only on alternate nights! We were used to bathing every day, though we soon adjusted to managing with the use of the hand basin in our room. What's more, it was expected that we should send our laundry out which would have been very expensive. This may have suited the English, but not us Aussies who changed our clothes every day and liked to dry them outdoors in the fresh air. To overcome this, we decided to wash our clothes in the basin and then hang them on lines we had strung up in the garden. Betty soon told us that this was forbidden as the house was on leasehold Crown land that forbade hanging washing outside. In this situation it was ridiculous, since nothing overlooked the garden and high wall. Next we rigged up lines in our room, which was also not allowed, though we continued to do so whenever we could get away with it. It was not surprising that cooking, even boiling a kettle was not allowed. To be fair I expect in London's bleak winters washing and steam could make the rooms very damp, but as all the boarders were well recommended the rules could have been less strict. We bought food for breakfast and ate from Aunt Jess's plates, while our other meals were eaten out.

Before leaving Australia we had been advised by our bank, The Bank of Australasia (now the ANZ), to contact their branch manager in London. We did so within a few days of our arrival, and the manager was most helpful in passing on useful hints as to places to eat at reasonable cost, the best sightseeing around London, and above all an offer of assistance if we had money or other problems. They were the days when banks actually cared and looked after the little customer, and when the manager greeted and knew all his customers. How things have changed! For more information, we contacted South Australia House, within The Aldwych at the end of The Strand. In 1952, any person going to London before leaving Australia was encouraged to join The Victoria League, which offered activities and assistance in many ways, including invitations for weekend stays in the homes of UK members. The League had clubrooms not far from Buckingham Palace, where members could drop in for tea or coffee and a snack, join in activities, read newspapers, and catch up with news of their homeland with other members from the colonies. We were very much a part of The British Empire and proud of it.

Jobs for Rae and Me

We quickly made the most of living in London by seeing as much as possible. Our priority was to find employment and so secure our futures with an income. As luck had it, dear Auntie Jess scoured the London newspapers and alerted me to an advertisement, which seemed ideal, promising not only employment but also accommodation and all meals. It was at The Strand Palace Hotel, in the Strand, right in the centre of London and almost opposite The Savoy. Not as exclusive as the latter but one of three quality establishments owned by The

A QUALITY LIFE

Lyons Coffee Houses Group. I applied for the position of Information Clerk and after a long and demanding interview with the lady Personnel Officer, I was accepted. Rae was equally lucky in quickly obtaining employment, a live-in teaching position at a Welsh girls boarding school near Windsor, where I believe she was very happy for the next five years that she was in England. Windsor had a regular and fast train connection to London which enabled her to visit often for day trips, theatre or special events, and so we continued to meet weekly and sometimes also for night outings.

Backpacking

After a few weeks in London and with a few more weeks before commencing work, we decided to see a little of England and Scotland. We had joined the Youth Hostel Association before departing Australia, and with a view to hitchhiking to Scotland, we purchased sleeping bags, sheets and backpacks from the Association's shop in London. We planned to take a train to Stratford-on-Avon and then get on the road from there.

Shortly before our departure I spent a few days at St Albans, an ancient Roman city just an hour by train north of London, where Auntie Jess and her son John lived at the home of a second cousin, Captain John Donaldson (Skipper to his relatives), a bachelor and Mayor of St Albans for many years. Skipper had visited Australia twice in order to make contact with his relatives, and on his last trip he asked Auntie Jess, who was divorced from Uncle John, if she would consider going to London to act as his Lady Mayoress. He would pay all expenses, including John's education, and provide for her for the remainder of her life. This was proving an excellent arrangement for them both, and opened a wonderful and interesting life for Auntie Jess, who was presented at Court, and in her new role played hostess several times to the Queen on her visits to St Albans. Skipper had a large home and garden with a live-in housekeeper, daily help and gardener. Auntie Jess was free to play tennis, golf and bridge, to socialise and to travel with Skipper around the country and to Europe with Auntie Kath when she visited. John attended St Albans Cathedral School and went on to study architecture at university. Skipper was very well respected and held the mayoral position for well over twenty years.

Some thirty years after Skipper's death, the Managing Director of the British parent company of Laporte, the company with whom my husband Errol was working in Sydney, was visiting Australia. Mr Ken Minton lived in St Albans and when I mentioned my association with that city, he told me that he knew of Skipper and that people still paid tribute to him for his contribution as Lord Mayor. The British plant was located near St Albans and had recently sponsored the costly replacement of the clear glass in the Cathedral's Rose Window, damaged during the war, with stained glass. As Skipper was an alderman of the Cathedral for much of his life, Auntie Jess had previously installed beautiful hanging lights there in his memory.

Skipper, hearing that Rae and I were heading for Stratford, thought we would be walking in the Dales. He gave me advice and maps of walking tracks (like many British, he was a keen walker), but then was horrified at learning of our real intention to hitchhike and warned of all the risks involved. However, undeterred, we set off as planned, and arriving at our destination, Stratford, the town of Shakespeare, were delighted with its many appealing sights. We lost no time in visiting these places before walking up the hill to the Youth Hostel on the edge of town. In those days, Youth Hostels were simple establishments: bunks in dormitories, communal bathrooms, and kitchens where occupants provided and cooked their own food, cleaning up after they had finished. The hostel provided mattresses and pillows and we carried our own sleeping bags, sheets and towels. A few (fortunately very few) hostels, even in Scotland, had no running hot water, but we were young and our expectations were much lower so we coped and it was all a wonderful adventure. Hostels were closed from 10 a.m. to 5 p.m., which meant that we could not gain shelter between those hours. There were certain rules: one had to arrive on foot, not by car, as hostels were for walkers, and one had to depart by ten after cleaning chores. Hitchhikers were treated as walkers, for hostels did not know (or care) who accepted rides. We travelled with: two sets of the fabulous new lightweight nylon underwear and one nylon blouse (washed and dried on the bedrail every night), nylon nightdress (washed and dried during day when we stayed two nights), sleeping sheet, woollen jumper, woollen twinset, two warm skirts, three pairs of warm socks, and a warm waterproof jacket and sturdy shoes (previously worn for golf).

Our first experience of hostelling was comfortable and with high hopes, we set out on the road. I expected we would walk along beside the road and some kind driver would stop and ask us if we wanted a lift, but to my horror, Rae informed me that we had to thumb a ride. I retorted that I would not stoop to that and would rather return to London and pay my way. Eventually I listened to reason and gingerly lifted my thumb in a half-hearted way. Rae was more enthusiastic and after a number of knock-backs, we were picked up by a truck driver who took us a long way north. We were heartened, and I not so faint-heartedly, soon entered into the joys of thumbing a ride and the excited anticipation of the next ride.

We continued on our way north to Yorkshire, and then to County Durham where we visited the remains of a historic cathedral (or castle!). A few days later, we entered Scotland at Gretna Green, famous as a place where until 1969 eloping couples avoided English marriage law. Then on to Glasgow, which we found old, dingy and grey, with very crowded housing. No doubt the rain helped create this impression.

Leaving Glasgow we were given a ride by two young journalists in their open sports car. How we and our backpacks squeezed in, I do not know, but we had a lot of fun and I have a photo of the occasion. They drove us through Rob Roy Pass, with bracken and pink heather covering the hills on both sides, and to the foot of Ben Lomond. With their encouragement, they left us there to climb the mountain. Reaching the summit, we rested and ate our lunch while looking over the magnificent surrounding pink countryside. The well-worn track took us little more than three hours up and two hours down, which we thought quite an achievement without mountain climbing experience. We stayed in a hostel, a former castle on the banks of Loch Lomond, which conjured up thoughts of sighting a monster, but no such luck; doubtless, he was taking a holiday.

We reached Edinburgh at the time of The Edinburgh Tattoo and consequently the city reflected all that is Scottish; proud of their ancestry, the people and the streets were in festival attire and in a festive mood. The city, one of the finest in Europe with its architecture and history, is well worth visiting and to do so in August during The Tattoo is an added bonus. We wandered along the main street with its quaint shops, and found most interesting our tours of the castles, the very ancient Hollyrood and Edinburgh Castle with its huge courtyard in front: a magnificent setting for the Tattoo. We were able to get close seats or standing room to see various events, and were enthralled and stirred by the bagpipes and the whole Scottish atmosphere. It is highly probable that in 1952 the festival events were very Scottish with little foreign participation, whereas today it has become more of an Arts Festival with bands, groups and artists from all over the world invited to perform. In addition, today, it would be impossible to get seats at the last minute and as affordable to our pockets.

We took the opportunity to have a look at nearby St Andrews Golf Links, but as we had to be on our way, decided not to play a few holes and declined an invitation to go inside the clubhouse! Before leaving Edinburgh, I replaced my waterlogged shoes with a sturdy new pair of skin shoes at a most excellent price. Nine years later these shoes returned to Australia with me, and even made their way to Sydney eighteen years later, where they provided ongoing comfort on special golf and country outings for yet another twelve years!

On the road to Perth we crossed the Firth of Forth Bridge - another landmark from our history books. We accepted a ride with a gentleman who was going north via Aberdeen to Balmoral Castle, exactly our destination. Though the Queen was in residence she had not invited us to visit, however as we had heard that members of the Royal Family frequently walked in the nearby woods, we hoped to get a glimpse of a Royal or at least have a view of the fairy-tale castle - the childhood home of the Queen Mother, Elizabeth Bowes-Lyon. Our new chauffeur told us that he was Secretary to the Queen, and although he was very friendly, he did not amend the Queen's obvious oversight. We had to be content with a viewing of Balmoral from a distance.

Our next destination was John o' Groats, the far tip of bonnie Scotland, a bleak, craggy, isolated spot with nothing to hold one for long - or so we thought. Returning south via the west coast, we had vague hopes of crossing to the romantic Isle of Skye. Unfortunately the boat sailings did not fit our schedule, so with disappointment we abandoned the idea. We then proceeded south feeling very happy with all of our recent experiences of beautiful countryside, the people, the history and the hostels - occasionally in castles - where even a cold water shower did not detract, as the camaraderie of fellow hostellers more than made up for any discomfort. Many days we set off from the hostels in the misty light rain, typically Scottish, which we found quite delightful and refreshing. The generosity and friendliness of all our drivers was more than we had anticipated and the hitchhiking proved such a fun experience that we were already talking of our next trip.

From the north of England we returned by train to London. Rae went on to her school and I went to St Albans for a day or so before taking up my position at the Strand Palace Hotel.

Living at the Strand Palace Hotel

Fifty years ago, as in many countries, transporting luggage presented no problem since at all stations, terminals and wharves there were numerous porters and people to assist with baggage, no matter how big. Larger items, like trunks, were offloaded and delivered to the door at very little cost, and while porters were pleased with small tips, they had no expectations. As well, cabs and other passenger vehicles did not cost the earth. London was no different and these services were provided with impressive efficiency. I arrived safely with my cases at the employees' entrance, which was located in an adjacent service building. It was on a side street around from the hotel, and the upper floors provided accommodation for the live-in female reception staff. I was led to my bedroom and introduced to my roommate, a senior receptionist who was kind and helpful. The first night I fell asleep excited at the prospect of starting my new job, which seemed so perfect, only to be rudely awakened at one a.m. by the sounds of shouting and yelling, trucks revving and roaring, and much clashing and banging as if the building was collapsing in some major disaster. Wide-awake, I realised that the noise was coming from outside. The annexe overlooked Covent Garden Market where produce was being delivered and stalls were being stacked in preparation for the day's market. Very dejected I decided that this job was not for me, and although my roommate assured me that after a few nights I would not hear the noise, I was not convinced. However sure enough, after enduring five nights of torture, I slept like a baby. This proved to me that it is possible, given time, to sleep through anything.

Our shifts ranged from 6 a.m. to midnight so all the information clerks, with the exception of Diana Delaney and Freda our boss, lived in the annexe. An overhead covered walkway connected the annexe to the hotel and we went by lift and then stairway to our office, which was above the hotel foyer.

This was the start of a new life and the easiest job I have ever had. Living cheaply and right in the centre of the city was ideal for a single girl hoping to see all she could of London. All meals: breakfast, lunch and dinner, plus morning and afternoon tea, and supper if we desired, were supplied to us in the staff canteen. Our meals were the same as those offered to the guests - and with the same choice. Even for morning tea, we had a variety of Danish pastries, and at afternoon tea there was a vast selection of French pastries, chocolate éclairs, rich cream cakes and scones. Even better, while the guests paid for all they ate, we indulged ourselves without spending a penny! With accommodation and meals provided and no costs travelling to and from work, the pay of twenty-seven shillings was really like pocket money and sufficient to cover entertainment. I had plenty of clothes, unlike my English workmates who rarely had more than two outfits, one for work and one for going out.

The title of information clerk was really a misnomer as it entailed connecting calls to and from guests' rooms (there was no direct dialling in those days), or taking messages. When guests dialled our number for information regarding theatre tickets, train times or sights around London, we would put them through to the hall porter; room complaints through to the housekeeper; and accounts to reception and so on. We simply were a conduit to other services within the hotel.

There were about six shifts in a day during which we went to meals, and as all shifts overlapped by about two hours, the leader of our team always allowed us to go off an hour early. For instance if our shift was seven to two, we went to breakfast soon after coming on duty, then morning tea around ten, and often left for lunch at twelve after which we were free to go. So in fact, we worked less than four and a half hours of our seven-hour shift. The eight-to-three shift was much the same, when we left at one instead of three. Only one person started at six, and was alone until seven when three others joined her, and then three more at eight. With all the breaks for meals and teas, no more than four girls were working at one time. On the four-to-eleven nightshift, three went off at ten, leaving one person who came on at five and stayed until midnight. This very relaxed timetable was designed to suit Freda, our leader, who lived some distance from London. Of course, no one complained, and I could not believe my luck. With so much free time, I was able to explore London, go on country outings in the daytime, and attend theatre or concerts at night. At times the shifts allowed for two or three days off, or we exchanged with other girls who were always happy to do so.

The girls, whose ages ranged from eighteen to twenty-eight in the main, came from counties far from London and were attracted by the big city. They were all very nice and friendly, and took much delight in teasing me about my accent. Though I must say, as they all came from all over England they had a variety of accents, none of which was exactly BBC, some very unattractive to my Aussie ears. Anne, in charge of the cigarette booth, enjoyed telling me of Australians on leave during the war who always asked for Cry-ven Eye (Craven A) cigarettes. It always intrigued me that Freda who seemed unable to pronounce the letter 't' when speaking with her normal accent (l'ille bi' o' bu'er - little bit of butter), always put on the poshest accent, pronouncing that letter clearly when answering the phone. Her accent was somewhere northeast of London but I am not sure of which county.

We did not socialise outside of work, as they were not interested in seeing London, the theatre or travelling elsewhere. The ones who did not have family living nearby were more interested in meeting the American airmen and marines, who were spending leave in London and had plenty of money to spend on the girls. The older girls who had been 'around' encouraged the young new ones to join them with stories of the good times the Americans gave them. New to London and not knowing anyone, the younger ones were happy to do so and very soon were living the high life of dinner, nightclubs and overnight stays in hotels - plus the occasional weekend away. I was still corresponding with Errol regularly and that relationship was developing seriously, so I had no interest in meeting men. My priority was getting to know London and England with my girlfriends, and to get away to St Albans, which I did frequently.

Getting to know England

When we arrived in London eating out was very expensive, and after the sumptuous meals we had consumed on board, we naturally were constantly hungry and found it difficult to fill our stomachs. Consequently, we sought value for our money. We missed our morning cups of tea most of all, as we had no facilities in our room for making a hot drink. We yearned for the days of living at home where we could eat all we wanted, have a cup of tea whenever we desired, and not have to pay.

When we went into our first teashop for afternoon tea, the waitress put a platter of tempting cakes on the table. We were faced with a real dilemma, as we had no idea whether the price for tea and cake meant one cake or more. We did not want to risk being charged for several, but on the other hand, we did not want to leave any if the price included them all. As we felt it was unhygienic to pass on uneaten cakes to other customers, we decided the best course of action was to eat the lot, which was probably about two each. This was a bad decision, and our first lesson that the English did not share our concerns for hygiene as we were charged for all the cakes - and at a pretty hefty price! From then on we were very wary, but unfortunately one had to enter and sit down before discovering the prices in any establishment.

Although it was several years after the war, certain foods were still in short supply, namely, meat, eggs, butter and tea for which we had ration books. Fortunately, while living in the hotel, I was not directly affected. During the war we in Australia had rationing too for some foods and clothing, but things were back to normal soon after the war ended.

The bank manager had told us that Lyons Coffee House on the corner of The Strand and Piccadilly Circus had excellent value for money, and that you could fill your plate as much as you liked for a set price. A range of courses was set out in buffet style as is done today in bistros, but was very novel in 1952. While still living at York Gate, we lost no time in taking the bank manager's advice. One night before going to the theatre, we had plenty of time and were most anxious to at last satisfy our hunger. There was a choice for each course, which we ate like ravished tigers giving thanks for every mouthful. The main course did not escape our hungry eyes and once again we piled the food high, but as our stomachs had shrunk since leaving the boat, not surprisingly we were uncomfortably full. We could not eat another mouthful and sat hoping to diminish the pile in front of us, but no matter how we tried the plate remained full. I have never forgotten our disgust at our own greediness, and feeling that everyone was looking at us. In a time of shortages we did not want to leave plates of uneaten food, but eventually realising that we would miss the theatre, we had

The United Kingdom!

to give up the losing battle and swallow our pride and leave. As a result we both felt quite ill, and needless to say, we never returned for another meal. Besides, soon after we both had our meals provided.

Together with Rae, Jeanette, and other friends, days were spent touring the sights of London: St Paul's Cathedral, Westminster Cathedral, the Houses of Parliament, the Tower of London, Kew Gardens, Regents Park Zoo, Hyde Park, Hampstead Heath and numerous art galleries and museums. And by bus or on foot generally exploring the shops, streets, markets and pubs which all make up the city's rich life and history - both factual and fictional.

Beyond London within reach by train were Oxford, Cambridge, Windsor Castle, Canterbury Cathedral and Hampton Court. We visited the latter in the spring, and I was entranced by the bluebells covering the ground everywhere. A magnificent mass of blue, they grew wild among the woods and open grass. Many times since, Rae has reminded me that I was so ecstatic at the sight that I fell on my knees and went absolutely mad, picking bluebells until my arms were overflowing with them. I do not believe that there were any signs forbidding picking, as the flowers stretched forever and grew profusely in springtime: only a mad Australian would behave in such a way. No one challenged me and I returned to London loaded with my 'ill-gotten gains'. We loved the deciduous trees, the delicate greens of spring, glorious autumn colours and the beautiful tracery when bare in winter or when covered with snow. Deciduous trees were rarely seen in Australia then, but now they are frequently planted in the colder southern climates. England is noted for its beautiful countryside and we loved to walk through woods and hedged country lanes, and to wander around the quaint villages.

One day I remarked to Auntie Jess about the beautiful colours in the bark of a tree. She was overjoyed and said, 'Do you really see the red, purple, browns, greys and different greens in the bark? If so, you are the only one beside me who can see them. Everyone else and Skipper think I am completely mad when I comment on the lovely colours, as they only see the tree trunk as a dull brown or grey, never a blend of individual brighter colours. When I write in my letters home and rave about the beauties of nature, trees, flowers and sunset, they all think I am exaggerating and seeing things through rose-coloured glasses.' From then on, we realised that we were kindred souls with a very special bond between us, which existed until she passed away shortly before her one hundred and second birthday on 22nd September 2001.

Later in life when she was still able to see detail, she marvelled at the intricate designs and colours that made up the centres of flowers - even the common daisy. She truly had a sensitive and artistic eye, as well as rose-coloured glasses. When it came to people, she never had a bad word to say, in all the years I can remember.

We attended all the theatres, opera and ballet whenever we could, as tickets were available in The Gods for the incredible and very affordable price of one shilling. Such entertainment was new to us and we loved every performance we saw. The Gods, as the gallery was popularly called, was very high, but as all theatres were small still gave an excellent view of the entire stage. As most plays ran for a long time there was no trouble in obtaining tickets (even for Covent Garden), though on occasions we queued at the ticket office for last minute tickets. On rare occasions, we bought standing room, which we had to for The Proms at Albert Hall where we queued from about 4 p.m. A vast area was set aside for 'standing room' only because these concerts were so popular. We enjoyed the new experience of queuing, chatting to people, and the whole atmosphere of the concerts and the enthusiasm of the audience, singing along with the choirs and celebrating their pride at being British. Huge flags decorated the Hall, and the members of the orchestra and choir dressed in the colours of the British Empire. It was most moving with all the audience waving Union Jacks, singing Pomp and Circumstance, Jerusalem and Rule Britannia. Unbelievably, at the precise moment I was typing RB, I heard a few bars of it played as background music on television. Nowadays the concerts extend to nearby Hyde Park, where thousands gather with their flags and Union Jack hats, to sing, watch the giant televisions and participate as enthusiastically as those indoors. Now the audience goes more overboard adorning their entire bodies with Union Jacks in every imaginable way. These proms are now in some larger city parks in London. Just before Christmas, Sydney too has evening proms in the Opera House; attended by British ex-pats and monarchists they are as stirring as those in London are.

We also went to the then new Festival Theatre where we learned to appreciate classical music and to know all the instruments of the orchestra. The year I spent in London was a true education in both the classical and musical arts.

Art at St Martin's

I already had an interest in painting and drawing from Woodlands, and later at Burra High School where Mr Eason saw some ink portrait drawings and encouraged me to continue. In those days, art was not seriously considered a vocation but rather as a leisure pursuit. London presented the ideal opportunity for me to receive some instruction. A fellow workmate, Hazel, expressed a desire to do the same so we decided to enrol at St Martin in the Fields, the then best known art school in London, I believe. The fees must have been quite modest and we were able to enrol in drawing and painting, one week attending day classes and the other weeknight classes, which suited us admirably. In the day drawing class, we went outdoors to parks, where there was a treasure trove of buildings and scenes waiting to be sketched. The Art School was very near the church of the same name and Trafalgar Square, so it was very close to the hotel. We had enrolled in a Portrait Painting in Oils class, and as neither of us had used this medium or knew how to approach the task ahead, we naturally expected some sort of instruction. None seemed forthcoming so we faced the board and easel with some trepidation, looking from left to right hoping to get tips from the other students. At the end of the 'lesson', the 'instructor' went around, looked at our work and offered criticism, but no useful advice as I recall. Despite this lack of assistance, we both produced a passable likeness of our models.

When finished, our paintings were taken to our hotel and placed around the limited space of our tiny rooms. I had since acquired a single room due to my new status of senior clerk. With a room to myself, I was able to spend my leisure time painting, and as my room was high rather like an attic, it provided good light. As a result, there was the constant smell of oil paint in the room, which added to the romantic notion of an artist's studio. No doubt, this contributed to our desire to move to Paris to pursue further studies in a bohemian atmosphere, more conducive to artists. Unknown to me at the time, many Australian artists had trodden this path to Paris and Montmartre, and gone on to be very successful. Who will ever know how different our lives may have been had we taken this step. My correspondence with Errol had continued with serious plans about being together in the near future, and so love conquered all. I don't know what happened to Hazel, but no doubt she too succumbed to love and marriage.

The Beaufort Hunt

One weekend after accepting an invitation via The Young Victoria League, Jeanette and I took a very early train to a village near Bath where we were met by our hosts Sir William Bt (Baronet) and Lady Wrixon-Becher. They were probably in their late thirties and a very natural and friendly couple. We later learned that Lady Wrixon-Becher's mother was a Lady-in-Waiting to the Queen Mother. He was a very keen cricket follower, and had accompanied the English cricket team to Australia once or twice so knew the country reasonably well. On arrival we were shown to our room, and when Lady Wrixon-Becher remarked, 'I expect you have eaten on the train', we were too polite to say that we had not. No doubt the Bechers always ate on the train, but that was an indulgence we could not afford. Had we told her we had not eaten, food would have been forthcoming immediately but we were too shy. The house though large was not grand, and all was very informal; we were made to feel very much at home. They were genuinely interested in us, our families, Australia and our future plans. So informal were they that both Jeanette and I were shocked to see jam served at Sunday breakfast without jam spoons or butter knifes. Such an observation may seem ridiculous to many of the present generation, but in Australia at that time and England too I believe, dipping one's knife in the jam pot was unacceptable to any well-bred person, as it still is to many of us.

A royal and busy weekend was ahead of us, starting soon after we arrived. Together with the Bechers' only daughter, Lady Alexandra Bridgewater, we all set off for the small village of Oldbury-on-the-Hill. She was a lovely girl, about fourteen years old, who may not have been Sir Williams daughter as her surname was not Becher. To me this implied she was a Lady in her own right. The Beaufort Hunt point-to-point race was held annually and attended by royalty and the aristocracy. In attendance were the Duke of Beaufort and a Maid of Honour for the Coronation, Lady Moyra Hamilton. This was a special coronation year event and people came from far afield. We all sat on rugs on the ground eating a picnic lunch, courtesy of the Bechers, and from time-to-time different titled people joined us for a chat. To our surprise, a photographer came by and took a group photograph for The Tatler, the English magazine reserved for the aristocracy, rich and famous. What an unexpected thrill for two Australian country girls!

I must say that those whom we met were all very down-to-earth, chatty, and welcoming despite our accent! I digress to say this because Betty Wylie had once commented to Auntie Jess, 'June is very nice but if she could only get rid of that awful accent.' Auntie Jess was very upset, particularly as Betty had been married to an Australian and had entertained numerous visitors with that same dreadful accent. The longer I stayed in England and later in Canada, the more I came to appreciate how the Australian accent sounded to English ears. It is interesting as I was always told that I did not have a very marked accent, and very often was asked if I was English. Perhaps I acquired this after a year's exposure to the British!

A few weeks after our weekend with the Bechers, we were thrilled to see the photograph taken at Oldbury-on-the-Hill in the society pages of The Tatler (25th March 1953) - a reminder of a very enjoyable weekend and our touch with the aristocracy.

A very nice gesture on the part of Lady Becher followed, as Mum reported that she had received a letter from her saying how much they had enjoyed our visit, and not to worry about me, as I was well and happy. Jeanette's family also received a letter.

Other days out of London included a visit to the beautiful city of Bath, the city of York with its magnificent York Minster and Roman Wall. The Farnborough Air Show is especially memorable, as there was the excitement of seeing the sound barrier broken and the tragedy of one plane crashing before our eyes.

That was a long day and we returned by train to London, Jeanette getting off at Ealing where she shared a flat, and Rae transferring to a Windsor-bound train once we arrived at Victoria Station. It was one a.m. when I discovered no buses were running, and as I only had one shilling in my pocket, I had no choice other than to walk. I set off along the Thames embankment and was approached by a policeman, who asked what I was doing out so late on my own. After I explained he obviously thought that I was no 'lady of the night' nor in any danger, and as I was not too worried I continued on my way. No one else approached me, nor did I see anyone. I can't imagine the undesirable characters I might encounter today or what fate might befall me. It shows how things have changed, not only in London but all over the world in every city and country.

When I wrote home telling of the above episode, I received a very concerned letter from my Mother scolding me for not carrying more money for a taxi should an emergency arise.

Visiting Jess and Skipper at St Albans

The many days and weekends at St Albans were very special with Auntie Jess and Skipper. Though very kind, Auntie Jess always said that he thought women were rather inferior to men, but I believe that as a long-standing bachelor he was shy, and being a highly intelligent, successful, well respected and a much-travelled man, that he came across as being superior. He had a great fondness for Auntie Jess, and welcomed to his home all his relatives and Australian cousins - no matter how distantly related.

His home, Kenmure, at 44 Sandpit Lane was a huge, comfortable, three-storey house with a large garden and tennis court. Kenmure had been the name of his home in Scotland, and Grandfather also chose that name for 8 Broadway in Glenelg.

At Kenmure, St Albans, the spacious entrance hall led into dining, sitting, study and powder rooms, which, together with a kitchen, pantry and scullery, were on the ground floor. There were four bedrooms and two bathrooms on the second floor, and at least two more rooms on the third including a bedroom for Elsie, the housekeeper, and another bedroom for John Miller, Auntie Jess' son. Above this, a steep stairway led to an attic study, where John studied and played his classical music, a pastime that provided enormous pleasure throughout his life.

His study was forbidden territory and it was a privilege to be allowed in. One day I was invited to enter to listen to his latest record of Vivaldi's Four Seasons, my introduction to that wonderful music. Sadly, he died from cancer two years ago, pre-deceasing his mother who was then one hundred. When I visited Kenmure, John was studying architecture at university.

At the back of the house near the tennis court, there was a vast vegetable garden, strawberry patch and raspberry canes which produced a bountiful supply of delicious fruit, all of which Auntie Jess and I feasted on. The house and garden are no longer there, having been replaced by a block of flats, which now covers the entire property.

Whenever I stayed at Kenmure, I was very spoiled by Auntie Jess, who each morning rolled in the traymobile and gave me breakfast in bed - a treat I loved. While I ate she sat drinking coffee, and we chatted about all and sundry. She recounted to me that when she and Auntie Kath went to the Continent, as it was referred to in the late forties, they had travelled by train. As it was shortly after the war there was still food rationing, and no food or drink was available at the stations. They carried sandwiches and a Primus stove, which they set up on the platform to make coffee while waiting for their next train.

She was both a friend and mother to me, and as we had so much in common, we enjoyed the opportunity to talk as only females so far removed from their family and native land can. She loved the countryside of England, the woods and beauty of the trees in all seasons, marvelling at the sudden burst of springtime, the green cool canopy of summer, the glorious autumn colours, and the cold starkness of winter relieved only by the mystery of fine shadows thrown on a blanket of white snow. I thought I had never seen such beauty. She was delighted when I told her that as a child, if I were to be reincarnated I wanted to come back as a tree, or so Fuff had told me. Auntie Jess fully empathised with such a desire.

Often with John at the wheel, Skipper took us on many excursions: to the beautiful Lakes District, the famous Whipsnade Zoo, and for a weekend sailing in his boat on the Norfolk Broads. What a pleasurable, lazy and fascinating experience, watching Skipper as he manoeuvred the boat along the canals and then through the locks.

On these outings we often took one particular picnic basket, which I have inherited by way of Auntie Jess. On Skipper's death, she was the sole beneficiary of all his household possessions, including his magnificent antique furniture, piano, sterling silver and more precious and mundane things. She returned to Australia bringing all with her, and was reunited with John, who had returned a few years earlier and since married Cathy.

At St Albans, domestic help was supervised by Elsie, their live-in housekeeper. Elsie was English and very efficient, and she had been seconded from Grandfather's house in Australia where we had all known her.

Originally, Elsie had come to Australia to be near her sister, and found live-in housekeeping at the Bryant household at No. 8

Broadway, Glenelg. Prior to her arrival there was daily help, but it was decided Auntie Kath needed more assistance as the home was so large. After all Grandfather was now less active (not that he did anything around the house), and I was living there too. Elsie performed her house duties conscientiously and reigned supreme in the kitchen. So much so that she watched my every movement like a hawk, especially when my friends came after school and we wanted milk and biscuits. She would allow only cordial and one biscuit each, ignoring Auntie Kath's instructions. She was a typical spinster, and played the role of housekeeper to perfection as if in a stately English home. She was definitely in charge of the household. She was loyal and very much a part of the Bryant family.

Skipper, when visiting Australia, had met Elsie and on learning that she wanted to return to England, offered to pay her fare and to employ her when Grandfather no longer needed her. This came about after Grandfather died and many of us resumed our relationships with her later in England.

John Miller, when aged nine, had numerous battles with Elsie before leaving to join Skipper in England. After yet another battle, I recall going for a walk with him and his tearful outburst, saying over and over, 'I hate Elsie, I hate Elsie, I hate her!' I wonder how he reacted when they met again a few years later! No doubt the situation was different, as his mother then became mistress of the house and was very protective of her only child. I was ten years older when Elsie and I met again and we greeted each other like family. We really were very fond of one another.

Girlfriends

Although they were much younger than I was, Diana Delaney and Julia were my special friends at the hotel. Diana was eighteen and lived with her family in a flat, just across the Thames in Rotherhithe. She was a very clever girl who should have gone onto higher education. One Sunday she invited me to her home for dinner. The small flat was rather crowded as Diana lived with her parents, a younger sister, a younger brother and Mrs Delaney's mother. They were a close Catholic family and it seemed to me that apart from work, Diana's life revolved around her family.

After Diana's sister and brother married, her parents relied solely on her. By then she had left The Strand and started working closer to home as secretary to the owners of a timber mill, where she only mixed with her bosses. It is not surprising that she never married as she would have met few young men, or so I believe. After many years of working, she bought a house in Kent for the family, and a car for herself. As her brother and sister grew up, married and had children, they became a major part of her life. It is sad that she has no family of her own, as she was a lovely, attractive girl with striking red hair. The remarkable thing about Diana is that for the fifty years since our Strand Palace days, every Christmas, wedding anniversary and birthday I have received a card from her, as have our three children for the forty years and more since their births. As well, she has kept similar contact with all our former workmates, including girls who married Canadian and American marines whom they had met on blind dates. Some of these girls who moved to North America, she has seen again when they have returned to England, and even now corresponds with their children. The cost of cards and postage over the fifty years must amount to many thousands of dollars. I once suggested that she could easily fund a visit to USA and to Australia. Unfortunately this has never come about, even though her oldest school friend has lived in Sydney for many years. Diana obviously enjoys keeping in touch this way, which is wonderful for the recipients. When we visited England with our children, she met us briefly and gave them a generous gift of five pounds each. Years later, when Ross was living in London he saw her again. Now we get an occasional email in addition to the regular letters and cards.

Julia, my other very special friend, came from working in a Brighton hotel to join us about six months before I left. A very beautiful nineteen year old, she was engaged to Cedric, a Frenchman, whom she met when he and his mother stayed at the hotel in Brighton. She was very romantic and madly in love with her fiancé, almost to the point of obsession.

I never met Cedric and I know one should not judge a person by his looks but he was a most strange looking man (from his photograph). No one could call him good-looking, but Julia thought he was the most handsome man in all the world and that she was very lucky. To my mind he was the lucky one, as she had the loveliest personality one could ever imagine. For some reason she liked and wanted to befriend me, maybe as a mother figure, and perhaps Cedric was a father figure as both her parents had died. Each night she turned back my top sheet and placed a chocolate on my pillow, as she did for her roommate. Before long, she invited me for the weekend to stay with her elder and only sister in Nottingham. Both her sister and architect husband were particularly friendly and ensured that I saw as much as possible in so short a time. We drove to Sherwood Forest, which I think no longer exists as such, though I believe it did in 1953. My memory is very hazy on that. We saw Nottingham Castle and spent some time in a very old pub made famous by Robin Hood, and with a name reminiscent of that era. The couple had two small children and because the spare room had just one double bed, Julia and I had to share, which we did not mind at all. I had grown up sharing a bed in such circumstances; besides it was a lot of fun as we talked long into the night - just as we had done in our childhood. The weekend went all too quickly and we boarded the train with sadness, but with an invitation for me to please visit again.

Plans to marry

Around this time, I was making plans to go to Canada to marry Errol. However in the years since then Errol has denied that he asked me to actually marry him, but to go to Canada to share his flat as his Australian friend was getting married and moving out. Errol's denial simply did not ring true, as those were the days when it was not acceptable for unmarried couples to live together. Besides, Errol was too moralistic to even consider such a thing, nor risk losing his job.

Back then, no reputable company would knowingly employ anyone living in sin.

The Coronation of Queen Elizabeth

The date for the Coronation of Queen Elizabeth was set for the 2nd June 1953, and as the date drew nearer, Auntie Jess said she would apply to Australia House for seats along the route that the procession would take. A certain number of seats were made available to citizens of each of the British colonies. She was successful in obtaining excellent viewing seats for the two of us, right opposite Westminster Abbey. In the following weeks tourists, especially Americans, flocked to the United Kingdom for the spectacle of a lifetime. The Americans were enthralled by the British Royal Family and this was an opportunity to not only be present at a historic event, but to view regal pageantry at its best. All London was abuzz with preparation for the occasion.

Of course, I was very excited at the prospect of being present, and as none of my workmates was fortunate enough to have seats, they willingly swapped shifts without any discernible envy.

The big day arrived. Auntie Jess came to London by train and I walked to our appointed meeting place and then on to our seats by seven a.m. We had around four hours to wait but time passed quickly as we watched the crowd and officials. During this time there came over the loudspeaker, the exciting news that the New Zealander Edmund Hillary and the Nepali Tenzing Norgay, had reached the summit of Mt. Everest. They were the first men to do so - another historic moment! From memory, we were ideally placed on about the third tier of the temporary stands that lined the entire route from Buckingham Palace to Westminster Abbey. We could not have had a better view had we been royalty. In fact, all the Royals inside the vast Abbey with its many columns would have had a very restricted view or no view at all of the actual crowning ceremony. By comparison, we saw the entire procession with commentary over loudspeakers, which commenced with the armed forces and police from Britain and all the colonies, Sherpas from Nepal, Canadian Mounted Police, Australian

Light Horse, Bags and Drums and so on. As well there were the Grenadier, Irish and Scots Guards and the various Queen's guards, both foot and mounted. Invited guests arrived in the order of least to most importance: commoners, politicians, aristocracy, representatives from all over the world, Prime Ministers, Heads of State and Presidents. Penultimately came royalty from Europe, the Middle East, Africa, and Asia dressed in their splendid and exotic robes. The huge smiling Queen of Tonga in her carriage was a magnificent sight.

While the procession was passing by I was busy scribbling all that was taking place before our eyes, so I could send a full account to my parents describing all the excitement, pomp and ceremony of this momentous occasion. My letter to them was published in the weekly Burra Record, a copy of which I still have.

At the exact moment of writing this, 10th April 2002 (9th April in Britain), another moment in history is taking place. The funeral procession of the Queen Mum, Elizabeth the Queen Mother, wife of King George VI (who died in 1952) is making its way through London to the service in Westminster Abbey. The much-loved Queen was one hundred and one when she died ten days ago. While her body was lying in state, four hundred thousand people lined the streets and came to mourn her passing - a record number on such an occasion.

Despite what many people think, I believe that the monarchy holds the country together, and without it, Britain would fall apart. It is the monarchy and all the associated pomp and ceremony that the tourists come to see, and that is the real money earner. On ceremonial occasions the Brits, even the Republicans, come out in full force and are proud that Britain can show how well they do it.

Preparing for married life

I had booked a flight to Canada in early July, which I was forced to cancel when I received an invitation (actually 'a command') to a Presentation and Garden Party at Buckingham Palace. No one could refuse the Queen, and who would want to miss such an opportunity?

Following this cancellation, I was faced with the problem of getting to Montreal. Everything by sea and air was heavily booked, owing to the number of North Americans wanting to return home after the Coronation. However, one day soon after, I received a phone call from the travel agent telling me that they had a seat at 1530 hours on July 19th. The confirmation of this flight arrived by mail a few days later. I was very excited and contacted Errol who then set in motion plans for us to be married on 20th July, the day following my arrival.

Accompanied by Auntie Jess, I had already been shopping for my trousseau (as all brides-to-be did in those days) in Kensington, a most exclusive shopping area, where I had bought a beautiful embroidered, off-white, calf-length Swiss-cotton frock; a lovely blue nylon frock with knife-pleated skirt (also calf-length); other day frocks and glamorous nylon underwear. The first nylon that was manufactured was very delicate and sheer so all frocks were lined. Shopping was a lot of fun but after a full day Auntie Jess declared that she was so tired, she could not walk another step. Being young I could not comprehend this, but as I grew older I fully understood! I wanted to buy a grey melange suit with a jacket and two skirts, one pleated and the other straight. Although such suits were in fashion, it proved very difficult to find one with two skirts, in grey and in my size. I tried Selfridges, the fashionable Harvey Nicholls and, to my delight, eventually found one in an exclusive shop in Oxford Street that specialised in suits. When I showed my purchases to Skipper, he quickly pointed out that one skirt was not the exact shade of grey as the jacket. I was amazed as neither Auntie Jess nor I had noticed the difference, and so the suit was returned. Finally, I found exactly what I wanted in a small shop in St Albans!

To complete my trousseau, Auntie Jess sewed by hand and smocked a beautiful nightgown and matching negligee in cream satin trimmed with lace - a treasured wedding gift from my darling aunt, which I still have to this day. And so, I was all set to be married.

Two weeks before flying to Canada, I left my work and friends at The Strand Palace. I was very sad to leave, as it had been a happy home and work environment for the past year. All the girls and I had had lots of fun and had become good friends. They seemed as sorry as I was to say farewell and presented me with a wedding gift of a set of serviettes, each one embroidered with different Royal Arms. These I still use together with the set of placemats and coasters with reproductions of famous architectural landmarks of London, a gift from Skipper. By coincidence, Rae also gave me a matching tray, which was much used but is no longer with us.

From the hotel I went to St Albans to spend time with Auntie Jess and Skipper, and to organise myself for my forthcoming marriage. I spent much time sorting out my trunk and repacking a case with clothes for our honeymoon. It was the custom not only to have wedding and going-away outfits, but to have mostly new clothes so the new bride would look her best for her new husband and he would be proud of her! At least he would not have to buy her clothes for a year or so, which I think was the main reason.

Around this time, Julia was to be married in Nottingham. She had asked me to be her bridesmaid, which I declined, as there was so much happening in June and July. Later I very much regretted my decision, as Julia was such a dear friend. Unfortunately, soon after my arrival in Montreal, she departed for Paris and we lost touch with each other.

A Royal Garden Party

A few days before the Garden Party all the presentees, about forty young girls from the colonies, were requested to go to Lancaster House in the Mall where a Lady-in-Waiting instructed us on how to curtsy and in what to expect and do on this Royal occasion. I had received a letter from a photographer offering a sitting and one free studio photograph, which required me to go to his studio after leaving the Palace. I had mine taken but unfortunately did not take up the offer - though I still have the proofs. Errol said he could take better photographs but that would not have been the same as a photograph taken on the actual day. Despite thousands of photographs since, there are surprisingly few formal portraits among them.

July 18th arrived. Dressed fit for royalty, in my summery Swiss cotton frock, hat and gloves, I took a taxi with Barbara Begg, another South Australian, up The Mall and through the gates of Buckingham Palace. As our taxis arrived we were ushered inside (not through the Royal front door used by the Queen) and into a great long hall. We, the presentees, were seated along the sides and after the ceremonial preliminaries were instructed to stand. The Queen entered and was escorted to her throne, on a dais at one end of the hall. We remained standing during the playing of the National Anthem, after which we all sat down again. Then as our names were called, we were escorted one at a time down the middle of the hall towards the throne, and from a distance of a few metres, we were announced. We nervously curtsied to Her Majesty, who graciously acknowledged. Still facing the Queen we stepped aside, then turned, and walked back to our seats. I for one, felt very thankful that I had not stumbled.

Afterwards we were ushered outside to the gardens where many other guests were gathered. This was the first garden party since the Coronation, and many dignitaries, who were in London, had been invited. We young girls were most fortunate to attend both the ceremony inside the Palace and the function outside in the gardens. I believe it was the last time that a Presentation ceremony for debutantes was held at the Palace.

In the gardens, a huge marquee was set up where afternoon tea was served with little sandwiches and the customary strawberries and cream. I think strawberries and cream still are standard fare for summer garden parties, not to mention Wimbledon. In Burra, they were always a special treat served with delicious clotted cream at St Mary's Church garden parties and at Red Cross fetes.

After partaking of afternoon tea, we wandered freely around the large gardens and lake, and mingled with the crowd. The Queen and Prince Philip chatted to various guests though I was not singled out. I was, however, next to a man whom Philip obviously recognised (perhaps his equerry reminded him) as he commented, 'I have been wanting to talk to you.' Although I have now forgotten the

THE UNITED KINGDOM!

conversation, I was most embarrassed as I could not avoid eavesdropping and I feared that the Duke might address me next. I was most impressed by his very natural and down-to-earth manner, as I felt sure that he did not know this man well but wished to make him feel at ease.

At the hour of departure, when the Royals retired, we regretfully left. I took one of the many taxis to the nearby photographer's studio, after which I returned to St Albans by train. The day's events left me feeling very excited and privileged.

I missed my flight!

My last two weeks in England slipped by happily and quickly. Skipper, who was very thorough and never left anything to chance, had insisted on checking my ticket. On the day of the 19th, he allowed two hours spare before my flight departed. In those days roads were not busy, and unlike today, one did not have to be at the airport hours before. Skipper, however, was of the view that if someone had not arrived fifteen minutes before the appointed time, then that person was already late. I recall the day when he had invited me to join him and Auntie Jess at a special meeting at the prestigious and ancient Guildhall in London, of which he was a member. This was a rare occasion when non-members could be invited. As later reported by Auntie Jess, fifteen minutes before I was due Skipper was constantly looking at his watch and declaring that I would be late. When I did arrive in good time, he still acted as though I was late!

It was a few minutes after three thirty when we approached the airport departure desk and Skipper handed the clerk my ticket. The clerk looked at the ticket and said, 'Sorry Sir, that plane has just left.' Skipper in his dignified way replied, 'It can't have, my niece is flying to Canada to be married tomorrow.' The response was, 'It left at three-thirty Sir.' Skipper then said, 'Her plane departs at five-thirty.' Then he looked at the ticket that he had previously checked so carefully, and saw 1530 hours. He could not believe his stupidity for he of all people, having been in the Navy, was familiar with the twenty-four hour clock system. Although I was aware that it was used in wartime, it was not common in peacetime. In truth, for weeks prior I had told everyone that my flight was July 19th at 5:30, and Skipper's mistake was that he, and everyone else, had been brainwashed by me. Skipper, however, could not accept this and blamed himself entirely. My excuse was that I was so excited when I received the phone call, that the agency had secured a seat on a flight departing 1530 July 19th, I translated it then as 5:30. This remained in my mind so when my ticket arrived, I really did not look at it properly and incorrectly read the time as 5:30.

Skipper asked the departures clerk if there was any other flight going to Montreal. The clerk was doubtful but said he would try if we would wait. To our surprise, within half an hour he returned with the news that there was one seat on a plane going via Iceland, departing shortly. It would arrive in Montreal an hour later than the other. I could not believe my good fortune. We sent off a telegram to Errol advising him that I was delayed, and of the changed arrival time. Then followed photographs, sad farewells, and for me the excitement of what lay ahead: the journey, marriage and a new life in a new country. Dear Auntie Jess was as excited as me, having already offered me advice on avoiding the mistakes she had made, for she blamed herself for her own failed marriage. According to my mother and aunts, it was the other way round, as Uncle John was very selfish, and she was very loving and worshipped him. I once asked had she ever considered marrying again, as I could see on my visits to St Albans that many men admired her. She replied that the only man she could have considered marrying, after John, was Earl Mountbatten!

From the moment the small plane taxied along the runway, I settled back to enjoy yet another new experience, my first overseas flight! And what an interesting route we were to take. How many people have been to Iceland, even today? There was so much to entertain me throughout the journey, from take-off to our landing in Ireland and thence north to Iceland in the Arctic Circle. As this was summer, the time of the midnight sun, the entire trip was in daylight. Some eight hours later we landed at Reykjavik airport, Iceland, where we all

The United Kingdom!

disembarked during refuelling. We passengers wandered around the small simple airport building set in a bleak flat country of large shallow pools, like lakes, of thawed-out snow. From the air, the small town looked desolate. In the air again over the North Atlantic Ocean, we headed towards the North American continent, then south over the heavily forested Labrador Peninsula and on to Newfoundland. This last part was most interesting. We all disembarked and went into the small building that served as the passenger terminal. Here I ordered a cup of tea and was startled when I saw the end of a string hanging over the rim of the cup. My first sighting of that American invention, the tea bag!

Finally, on the last leg to Canada and Quebec Province, our flight path followed the vast St Lawrence River south over Quebec City to Montreal, an island in the river. Mount Royal rises in the middle of the city, with the city proper stretching from the southern foot of the mountain and beyond to the St Lawrence River, which originally formed a natural city boundary. Of course, the city has long since expanded to the other side of the river. As we circled over the city, I was surprised at how small the city seemed for a population of one million. By comparison, Sydney covered a much larger area. Later I was to discover that Montreal was, in the main, a city of apartment dwellers. However, my view from the air revealed an attractive and unique setting for a city, which indeed it proved to be.

Canada - Reunited with Errol

It was almost twenty-four hours from take-off in London, to landing in Montreal at eleven thirty, on Sunday July 19th. Errol was anxiously waiting for me and one of his first questions was to enquire the reason for my delayed flight. Like a fool I told him, which was a mistake as I do have a tendency to run late. He has never let me forget, often reminding me by telling people that I was even late for my wedding! Of course that is not true, as my plane arrived shortly after the first booked flight.

From the airport we drove in Errol's two-seater coupe, which I thought was pretty snazzy, to the home of Ed and Inez McAsey in NDG (Notre Dame de Grace), a two-storey duplex where I was to stay overnight. Before going inside he presented me with a beautiful engagement ring, a large diamond with two small ones on either side set in white gold. The McAseys were good friends of Errol's and became dear friends of mine too. They had two children, Judy and Brian, and Inez's mother, Mrs Meagher, also lived with them. Mrs Meagher had another daughter, married to an Australian, whom she had visited in Crystal Brook near Port Pirie, the town where Errol had worked with Broken Hill Associated Smelters before leaving Australia. After arriving in Montreal, Errol was introduced to the family by his Australian flatmate, who had met Mrs Meagher at the time of her Australian visit. They made me very welcome and I immediately felt at home. I had a long rest, as Errol's boss and his wife had planned a late afternoon party to celebrate our nuptials the following day.

The party was held at the home of Selby and Betty McLeod who lived in a new suburb on The Lakeshore, so called because the St Lawrence forms a lake at this point. About forty work colleagues from the Foundation Company of Canada and their partners were present. Their friendliness towards me, I felt, reflected their high regard for Errol and his popularity. Wearing my new blue nylon dress, I was very relaxed knowing that I was among friends. Immediately, I was aware of the marked differences between Australians and Canadians, speech and expressions, customs and even drinks. On being asked what I would like to drink, I replied a sherry, as that was the usual drink at that hour for women in Australia and England. Few women drank hard liquor, although Aunties Kath and Jess as long as I could remember had a brandy before dinner. As most people had sherry on hand, it was always a polite and safe choice. Not so in Canada, as sherry seemed an unusual request. I was soon introduced to Canadian rye (whisky) mixed with Canada Dry (ginger ale); a very pleasant drink, which from then became my favourite. Errol had been a teetotaller in Australia and although he would join his friends at the pub, he drank only lemonade. In Canada, however, he soon discovered a fondness for rye and for other alcohol in the years to come.

A Montreal wedding

An early night followed the party in preparation for our wedding the next day. As 20th July 1953 was a Monday, a working day, and none of our relatives were to be present, the ceremony was attended only by Errol's close friends as witnesses: the McAseys, the McLeods and Earl Younghusband who gave me away. We were married by Rev Canon Oliver in the chapel of St Matthias Church, Westmount, a beautiful old church just across a small park from Errol's apartment at 3025 Sherbrooke Street. Five and six years later, respectively, both our sons Trevor and Ross were to be baptised here by Canon Oliver. Only after our vows were made and the Register was signed and witnessed, was it realised that Errol, a keen photographer, had neglected to organise photographs. Earl made a quick dash to fetch a camera from Errol's apartment, and duly recorded the occasion. Following photographs we returned to the McAseys, changed clothes (incidentally, I had not worn the Swiss cotton frock as originally intended because I later found a brocade one in Kensington, which Auntie Jess and I preferred) and were soon on our way to Ottawa.

Honeymoon at Château Laurier

I was amazed by the beautiful country and the number of lakes, with every turn in the road revealing yet another one. Some were fringed with tall fir trees and lay between low mountains covered with Canadian maples, still in summer leaf but preparing to don their colourful autumn garb. In some sections of the road the trees met overhead, forming a long archway filtering the sunlight on to the roadway. The weather was ideal, warm and sunny. Two odd and silly things stand out in my memory: the frequency of Errol's stops for aerated drinks, and that whenever he spoke to me I had to say, 'I beg your pardon.' I don't know whether he spoke quietly, if it was the noise of the car, or that I was preoccupied admiring the scenery. Whatever the reason, his every remark from then on was preceded by, 'Calling all cars!' To this day we joke about it, and often when driving he alerts me first by using this phrase before continuing with his main comment.

Ottawa, the capital of Canada, has some magnificent old buildings. The most outstanding is Château Laurier, which, together with Le Château Frontenac in Quebec City, and Château Lake Louise and Banff Springs Hotel in the Canadian Rockies, are grand hotels built by Grand Trunk Railways at the end of the nineteenth century. This was the start to the honeymoon of every girl's dream, for here in the Château Laurier we spent our first night together. Our large room was decked with flowers as though awaiting royal visitors, overlooked trees, Parliament Square and Government House. We ordered dinner with champagne in our room and, after wheeling it in on a trolley, the two waiters set up a table by the window to serve us by candlelight with all the trimmings and protocol reserved for special guests. Breakfast followed much the same procedure the next morning - I was quickly learning the ways of royalty!

With great anticipation we set off, keen to see more of this beautiful country so different from our homeland. We left Ottawa for our next stop, Algonquin Park, where Errol had booked three nights in a log cabin beside Joe's Lake. We threaded our way between mountains and more lakes, small and large. To my mind this seemed typical Canadian country as one imagines from films: log cabins set amongst giant firs at lake's edge, all reflected in the still water, small canoes pulled on to shore and, perhaps, a jetty where larger craft could cast off. This was even more beautiful than any of our expectations, as the lake disappeared into the distance between the mountains and all was peace and solitude. Nowadays some lakes are no longer peaceful, with powerboats and jet-skis thrashing through the water. Hopefully, Algonquin being a National Park has escaped such a fate.

We loved our comfy cabin, lying in bed listening to the squirrels clambering over the roof and to the birdcalls breaking the dawn. We relaxed, went for walks in the woods, lazily rowed the little canoes on the lake and adjourned to the main lodge for tasty meals. We were sorry to leave Algonquin but our next destination was Niagara Falls, which reigned as the honeymoon capital of the world, long before Hawaii became popular. Today couples choose from a greater variety of destinations, whimsically exotic or not.

Even miles from Niagara, or so it seemed, we could hear the deafening roar of rushing water. What an exhilarating sound and sight it was, this massive expanse of water thundering down to the swirling, bubbling pool far below!

Once again, Errol had excelled himself by booking us into the General Brock Hotel, immediately opposite the river and falls. Our room on the top floor had an excellent view of the floodlit Horseshoe Falls on the Canadian side. The American Falls, across the border by way of a bridge, are not as spectacular. After checking in, we hurried out to a get a closer view and to book tours for the following day. Each night when seated for dinner by the window, and again later from our bedroom, we were surprised and delighted to see the falls in their colourful floodlit guise.

Despite the background of roaring water, we slept soundly, and after breakfast we left excitedly for our first tour. The Maid of The Mist ploughed through the heavy churning waters below the falls - an exciting trip following the flow of the Niagara, enabling us to view the canyon and falls from a different perspective. In the afternoon, covered from head to toe in waterproof gear with hoods and boots, we went underground by elevator and then through a tunnel to a rock platform right beside the foot of the Horseshoe Falls. To be so close, almost under the giant fall itself, was an exhilarating and scary experience. The noise was beyond belief; I think we may have worn earmuffs.

The next day we crossed on foot the bridge spanning the river to the American side of the township of Niagara, to view the American Falls, which can only be approached from the USA. This was not the tourist side as the main falls were in, and facing towards Canada. Here we were taken down the many steps in the rock face to rock platforms where we viewed the long falls and, though outstanding, they could not be compared to the Canadian falls. Back on Canadian soil, we hired a horse and carriage to take us a little downstream for a cable car ride across the vast river. To me at the time this was terrifying – held precariously above the turmoil, roaring like some prehistoric animal waiting to swallow us up.

More than thirty years later, we again visited Niagara from Toronto. We had intended driving ourselves but fortunately friends took us. When we arrived, it was so crowded it was impossible to park. There was no alternative but for Bunny and John Scholes to drop us off and go out of town to park, with the intention of returning within half an hour. We jumped out of the car and wended our way through the dense crowd for a quick look at the falls and a short walk, then back through the crowd once more to await the Scholes. There was no desire for us to stay longer; at least we had returned, disappointing though it was. We were so pleased to have visited in the days when it could be enjoyed.

After leaving Niagara and Ontario, in the second week of our honeymoon we drove south of the border into New York State. We visited Rochester, the home of Eastman Kodak, which Errol was very keen to visit. The comprehensive tour was enlightening, particularly to me and possibly to Errol also. When we were taken into a room lit only by infrared light, Errol asked me to hold his hand saying that he could not see - for all to him was pitch black. The rest of the factory was lit normally and he was able to enjoy the remainder of the tour. I was curious to know the reason for Errol's temporary blindness and he said that he was colour-blind. I was intrigued by this disclosure and as I had never known anyone with this affliction, I bombarded him with questions. For some days after I constantly asked him what were the colours of the cars we saw on the street; he became very cunning, often guessing red when in doubt. I could see the problems a colour-blind child might have in school, as often colours are indicated or objects are pointed out by colour, as in, 'see that red house', or 'the tree with the red flowers', or 'repeat and learn the passage written in red'. A person who is red-green colour blind can confuse these two as well as secondary colours like brown, which contain a combination of both. Strangely, he has never confused traffic lights as he can recognise the placement and a difference in hue. Nor has he ever put a wrong tie or shirt with a suit, although once he bought a purple tie and, very early in our marriage, was surprised when I referred to his two brown suits, both of which he thought were different shades of grey.

In the last days of our honeymoon, we drove slowly east through the New England State of Vermont and the Appalachian Mountains, staying overnight wherever we found appealing. We were entranced by the picturesque lakeside villages, and the beauty of the slender silver birches, deciduous trees and mountains. One place which particularly delighted us was Lake Placid, which had hosted the Winter Olympics a year or so before and did so again many years later. As we had done before we stayed in one of the many motels; these 'motor-hotels' were then completely unheard of in Australia. We had discovered that because of competition, the owners were prepared to settle for any amount rather than have an empty room, and that the nearer to a town the cheaper the rate became. We visited the hometown of Robert Louis Stevenson. In our wanderings there we came across a peach tree laden with luscious fruit, hanging over a fence, and could not resist the temptation to pluck a few. It was a light-hearted moment and as with children, there was a certain thrill associated with the guilty act, followed by the relief of not being caught ... even more embarrassing for adults.

As motels did not serve meals, we ate whenever we could at Howard Johnson's chain of restaurants that served excellent meals at low cost. They were famous for their highly advertised forty-four flavours of icecream. We were introduced to American apple pie, and also lemon meringue pie and pumpkin pie. The latter became a family favourite in the years to come, though on returning to Australia my father stubbornly refused to taste it, as pumpkin was a vegetable not a sweet!

Along the way we also frequented the roadside diners (tram-like structures with booth seating), popular with travellers where we found the very traditional Canadian and New England breakfast of pancakes and maple syrup served with sausages or bacon very much to our liking. One evening we ordered the popular T-bone steaks. We expected a large steak but were not prepared for the gigantic ones set before us. Tender and delicious though they were, we were able to eat less than a third of each.

Other novelties were that drugstores sold sweets and milkshakes, as well as pharmaceuticals, and that all orders came accompanied with a glass of water. The glass of water was also placed on the table when the customer sat down in any eating establishment, even when ordering coffee. In a few places, this healthy practice has been adopted in Australia, but in general, it is very rare to get waiters to bring water during meals, even after numerous reminders. So unlike Turkey, where even in the cheap lokantas a bottle of water is always put on the table and replaced as soon as emptied.

The last night of our honeymoon was spent by Lake Champlain, just below the border. As we were both landed migrants crossing into Canada, customs presented no difficulty the following day. We were required to fill in declarations and were allowed entry without being searched. There were limitations on certain items and we had heard stories of difficult officers who insisted on thorough searches thereby causing much delay.

A few hours later we approached the Mercier Bridge, the southern link to the Montreal Island and City. (The Jacques Cartier Bridge provided a northern crossing.) Fortunately, there was no traffic line-up as regularly occurred at weekends, when one could wait for more than an hour to get on or off the island. Over the years the problem has been overcome, I believe.

Our first home together

Within half an hour, we had arrived at our apartment on the third floor of 3025 Sherbrooke Street. On the corner of Atwater, it was on the boundary between the upmarket suburb of Westmount and the city. Sherbrooke ran the entire length of the island, from the western English suburbs to the East End and French Quarter. It was a beautiful tree-lined street with many public buildings, the Museum of Montreal, the Ritz Carlton Hotel, Magill University, professional rooms and office buildings, including The Foundation Company where Errol worked.

I was delighted with the apartment, our very first home. From the front door, a passage on the left ran the length of the apartment with the bedroom on the right, then the bathroom and small kitchen. The passage led into the sitting room with an archway to a dining room on the right, which had a doorway to the kitchen. It was quite roomy, and Errol and Colin (his former flatmate) had furnished it very well, including even table lamps, kitchen equipment and two dinner sets. In Montreal there were many wealthy people constantly updating their homes, so there were many bargains of good second-hand furniture to be had. Errol purchased a beautiful and rare Canadian maple bedroom suite: bed, two dressing tables, chests and bedside tables. We later regretted not shipping it to Australia. In the first few days, I found just one drawback, the apartment got no direct sun and only a little reflected from the wall of the adjacent building. Errol's reply to this was that, 'Some people do not even have windows.' All our rooms had windows but looked out onto walls; over time, this no longer worried me.

We had arrived on Friday, in time for the weekend, so on Sunday Errol suggested a game of tennis. I was dressed in my tennis clothes all ready to go when, to my surprise, Errol said that I couldn't go like that, as no-one arrived at the club dressed for tennis but changed there! Some years later when our friends Malcolm and Wendy Ferrier joined the club, they dared to break this golden rule. I had never heard of such a thing before, but rather than show my ignorance and disgrace my new husband, I dutifully changed back into my street clothes. On arriving at the Monkland Tennis Club, we met George and Dot Perry, newly married, who had just moved into our apartment block. George, a fellow Australian, was Errol's regular doubles partner. Errol left me with Dot, who introduced me just as June Burdon to Margaret Godwin. Marg took me down to the locker rooms and once again, I was introduced as June Burdon to other girls. I was shocked when asked if I was Errol's sister, and realised that no one had known of his coming marriage. He had made many good friends, some female, whom he had taken out almost up to the time of his marriage. No doubt they were more surprised than I was. When I asked Errol why he had not told anyone, he said it was no-one else's business. Errol is a very private person and I expect it is hard to suddenly announce that you are getting married. Ed and Inez were told about me, as they had introduced him to a number of girls, all of whom he had found lacking for some reason or other. Inez told me later that she had said to Errol that I must be pretty special, to which he replied, 'She is.'

Over the eighteen months we were apart, he had put me on a pedestal that was impossible to live up to. He was rather disillusioned that I was normal, with many imperfections. He had never lived with a woman in the house, apart from his older sister who had looked after him, his father and brother, Ivor. Errol's parents had divorced when he was still at school. In recent years, he had lived in bachelor's quarters in Port Pirie, and even when quite small he had done whatever he liked without having to consider anyone else. Consequently, he found it hard to accommodate a companion day and night. By contrast I found it strange, and very difficult to be in the company of someone who did not speak for hours. I had always been surrounded by talkative women, among them my three sisters and most recently my workmates. It was quite amusing when one day in the kitchen, I remarked that I had forgotten what I was doing. Errol was amazed at my comment, and when I restated, 'Well, I have forgotten', he could not believe it and thought I was losing my mind. He had never heard of it before, but it has happened to him on many occasions since!

Errol returned to work on the Monday following our honeymoon and gradually we settled into a busy and happy routine. Our life centred around the tennis club where we went most nights after work and I too made friends, the first being Marg and Yolan Gregor who were Errol's friends and became my regular tennis partners. All club members were friendly and made a close social group. Over time we had special friends: Ethel and Bryant Murphy, Claire and George Knight, the newer members Stella and Tony Bennett, and Wendy and Malcolm Ferrier for the time they lived in Montreal. Some were non-playing members, but together we still had lots of fun. After tennis on Saturdays, we met with friends at Chicken Charlies on Sherbrooke Street for BBQ chicken, French fries and salad, and rolls to soak up the generous serve of luscious gravy. Afterwards there were various dessert pies available; our favourites were cherry pie and Boston cream pie. Invariably we all chose the latter, which was not really a pie but rather a cake, a very light butter cake filled with about an inch of French vanilla custard and topped with chocolate icing. It was sheer bliss to eat, and served with icecream we never tired of it. It seems that this pie is unknown outside of North America and although I have tried recipes in American cookbooks, I have never achieved the right texture or flavour of the vanilla cream.

Ed and Inez were our family, inviting us to their home for Christmas dinner and other special occasions. For many years, they were always on hand when needed. They were keen bridge players and we often visited each other for dinner and a game of bridge. Other times we just played bridge followed by supper. Inez was a good cook and as I was just learning, I experimented and tried to do something special. They were devout Catholics and though Ed had studied for the priesthood (giving up due to ill health), he always appreciated an irreverent joke about the Catholic religion. Errol was forever telling such jokes and neither Ed nor Inez ever resented it. One night after bridge when I brought in supper, they announced that because it was Lent, Ed could not have anything to eat. Inez however, who was teaching at the time, argued she needed to keep up her strength and gleefully ate several cream puffs. We thought this hypocritical, even though the church had decreed that people in certain professions were exempt from fasting. Silently we wondered what nutrition cream puffs could possibly provide. In Quebec Province the Catholic Church was quite corrupt. In exchange for a donation, one could acquire a receipt for a hugely inflated sum ($2 earning a $100 receipt), thereby entitling the donor to an excessive income tax deduction. Surprisingly these receipts were readily available to non-Catholics as well, and a Frenchman from work once asked Errol if he wished to take advantage of the scheme. Errol declined the offer.

Settling in to Montreal

Within a week or so of settling into our first home, I was anxious to find some work me as everyone I knew was employed. Errol's office was only five minutes away and though he came home for lunch, the small apartment was not enough to keep me occupied.

The first job I applied for was as a bookkeeper and when asked what salary I was looking for I was completely thrown. Of course I wanted to say as much as I could get, but this was an unexpected question and unheard of in Australia. Somehow I managed to get around that dilemma, and in any case, I turned down the position, as the location was difficult to get to.

I then found a part-time job with an Egyptian family, newly arrived from Italy. They lived in one of the large, old Westmount homes, a few streets up the mountain behind our building. I was required to look after their four-year-old daughter, who already spoke Arabic and French, and some Italian as she had an Italian nanny. The rest of the family was also fluent in these languages, except the mother who had never learned Italian. Two older daughters were learning English at school, as was the father with his work. My job was to entertain and play with the child, speaking only in English for four hours each afternoon until her sister came home. Whenever the mother or the nanny came into the room, it was fascinating to see the four year old suddenly switch to French or Italian, and even translating for her mother what the nanny had said and vice versa. The ability of small children to learn several languages at one time is truly amazing. Even the older children in that family had no trouble with English, after only a few weeks of tuition. This job lasted only a short time. The child got bored with me hanging around, as I did too; besides, she was learning quickly from her sisters.

At that time in Montreal, English was the official language, and all business was conducted in English, despite the fact that two-thirds of the population were French. The majority of the French spoke excellent English, in particular because all government, business and shop positions required fluent English. I was constantly amazed that when a customer went into a shop, the assistant in some uncanny way knew instantly whether that person was English or French, and never failed to use the correct form of address. On the other hand, the English forgot all their school French, never bothering to use it unless they had grown up in a French quarter. Now things have turned the other way. Consequently, Montreal is no longer the business capital and all head offices have moved to Toronto.

The Bell Telephone Company was issuing a 5 per cent bonus on all shares, and advertised for a number of temporary employees for a six-week period to calculate the payout to each shareholder. We were seated at desks in a large room, and given a list of shareholders and the number of shares they held. We were also given sheets of tables showing the correct bonus amount for any number of shares. I quickly did away with the tables, preferring to work the answers out in my head and then write them down beside the name of the shareholder and his number of shares. It was quicker and easier than fiddling with two lots of sheets. After all they were using the decimal system, dollars and cents not pounds, shillings and pence. When the senior manager came around checking everyone, he was horrified to see what I was doing. He could not conceive how I could do it in my head. When I explained how simple it was by knocking off the last digit and halving he still did not understand, and insisted I refer to the tables as I might make a mistake. I said I was more likely to make a mistake lining up the number of shares in the table and then transferring, but all was to no avail. Errol and I were forever surprised at how little people understood the decimal system. In one shop, we encountered a man who was unable to figure out the cost of ten items at 99 cents each, and we soon became aware that this was not at all unusual. Unfortunately, now the same happens in Australia.

The Foundation Company was responsible for the set-up and construction of the Distant Early Warning radar system (DEW) in Canada's far north. DEW was designed to detect any approaching enemy aircraft or missiles from the Soviet Union. A new project team had taken over a floor of the building for extra administrative staff, and it was suggested to Errol that I might work with the team. For three months I was employed as an assistant to the boss's secretary, a position made as a favour I suspect, as there really was little to do. However as the staff were friendly and the atmosphere congenial, I was very happy to be there. It was an enjoyable period. Errol and I walked to work together, and had coffee and Danish pastries each morning in the coffee shop in the building.

While looking for further work I decided to continue my art studies and went to the Museum of Montreal Gallery where I was interviewed by the head of the art school, Dr Arthur Lismer. Dr Lismer was a delightful white-haired septuagenarian and one of the famous Group of Four, so named in the twenties for their outstanding paintings of the Canadian wilderness. He was interested to learn that I was an Australian, as in the 1920s he had spent some time teaching in

Melbourne. Impressed by my oil portraits from London, he promoted me to second year and gave me great encouragement. Under his instruction, I concentrated on figure and nude drawing - one of the basic skills essential to becoming a competent artist. At the end of the year, the school held an exhibition of student work at the Museum. I have a photo of me dressed in my elegant grey suit, standing on the museum steps holding my paintings, my attire a far cry from art student dress of today! People dressed more formally in those days, even on holidays, as illustrated by another photo of me in the same suit and high heels standing in front of The Capitol building when sightseeing in Washington.

When I found permanent employment at The Bank of Nova Scotia, I was sad to leave the stimulation and creative atmosphere of the art school. The bank on Greene Avenue, Westmount was less than ten minutes from home, which was ideal. I was employed as senior ledger-keeper, relief teller and for a time as assistant accountant. In Canada and in the USA, the tellers were young and inexperienced, and more like shop assistants dealing with money. In the fifties in Australia and I believe elsewhere in the world, tellers were senior bank officers with considerable responsibility.

I digress to tell of our experience when travelling around Turkey in 1991, where we stepped back in time in a town east of Adiyaman and Malatya. The town had several banks, and in the one we entered there were four distinguished gentlemen in the tellers' cages. Despite the dirt and dust outside, they were immaculately dressed in modern grey suits, white shirts and ties. Clearly, even in Turkey, it seemed the teller held a responsible and respected senior position. We were interested to see two beautifully dressed little boys in the bank, sitting sipping tea while waiting for their mother. In the same town we entered a chemist shop, to find the owner absent and two young boys in charge. While trying to demonstrate with sign language that we needed something for a sore throat, one of the boys insisted on going to fetch us some tea. After much laughter and searching through shelves, we finally departed sustained by the tea, content with our purchase and delighted by the friendly humour of the boys.

Early on apart from the tennis club and seeing the McAseys, we saw a lot of Selby and Betty McLeod who entertained us on their boat at weekends. They were very generous and lots of fun, and together with their young daughter, we spent many happy times on the lakes and canals of the St Lawrence River and Lake Champlain. The boat was roomy and comfortable, the lakes beautiful, and from time to time we berthed at various marinas, going ashore for meals or drinks. We met interesting people from Canada, the USA and elsewhere, some of whom were very wealthy with huge boats. These 'boaties' were very friendly and happy to show us over their luxurious homes away from home. Sadly, three years later this all ended when the McLeods were on the way to Florida for a vacation. Selby had a heart attack and tragically died, still in his mid-fifties. Errol was devastated, as Selby was not only a good friend but also a wonderful boss. Somehow, we lost touch with Betty when she later remarried.

Our first fall in Canada we were dazzled by the myriad colours, covering the countryside like a patchwork quilt with every imaginable shade of yellow, orange, apricot, peach, plum, wine, red and rust. Every year when we visited the Laurentian Mountains to the north, or the eastern townships of Quebec, Vermont and New Hampshire, we never ceased to marvel at the colours. Later too when the leaves lay thick on the ground, we experienced child-like joy at the dry crackling sound as we kicked our way through them. In the country, the smell of burning leaves was like incense filling the air.

Though tennis was not played during the colder months, the club remained open for social functions, bridge evenings or just get-togethers around the bar. Errol played bridge one night a week, but I did not feel confident enough to play duplicate, which in retrospect was a mistake. Ten-pin bowling was a very popular winter pastime and we both played in a tennis club team one night a week. It was great fun and occasionally we played with friends at the weekend. Errol took to bowling like a duck to water, and with his team from work achieved record scores.

Generally, the warmer months were the time for family vacations. For others, longer days meant opportunities in the evenings for outdoor pursuits, sport and gardening. Evening classes were held over the colder and winter months allowing me to follow some of my interests. After leaving the art school, I attended a portrait painting class with Eric Goldberg, another member of the Group of Four. It was a small class with a model and held in his home. I think it was quite expensive, as I gave it up after a while. Much later when I was pregnant with our first child, I attended evening French classes in one of the nearby schools, Cote St Luc, gaining a proficiency certificate, no doubt presented as a noble gesture for attendance - almost to the day the baby was born! When again pregnant the following year, I went to classes at the YWCA on downtown St Catherine Street. The study of pottery making, more often referred to as ceramics nowadays, was relatively unheard of as a hobby pursuit in the 1960s and I was fortunate to find a class run by a charming and knowledgeable older Austrian lady. I was fascinated with all aspects of the process: the kneading, the moulding or throwing, the painting, the glazing and firing to the finished creation. Although I took up the craft again later, I never really mastered the skill of wheel throwing, much preferring handwork. I still have many pieces from Montreal days, as well as those made years later.

Despite the extreme winters, the cold did not worry us. All buildings and trams were well heated, and we were rugged up when outdoors. Once the snow lay thick on the ground in mid-winter, the skies were clear and sunny and it seemed much warmer than the temperature gauge indicated. We loved walking in the snow and like children crunched it beneath our feet. I delighted in rolling in it! Mount Royal, so accessible, is a huge natural playground. It is popular for walking, cycling and riding all year round, and in winter people can ski and toboggan, and skate on the frozen lake. A highlight is to take a horse-drawn sleigh ride to the summit. There is a fine panoramic view over Montreal and the St Lawrence River, similar to the view one has from Mt Wellington of Hobart and the Derwent. Having said that, the St Lawrence River is on a much grander scale while Mount Royal is nowhere near as rugged or as high. In all seasons, we took visitors to the mountain. Though one could walk we never did, as it was a steep hike from our apartment.

As George and Dot lived in the same apartment building, we spent much time together including playing cards regularly. These evenings were always arranged at the last minute when Errol and George met in the foyer returning home from work. After a year or more of playing, one night Errol came home and said George had commented that we had not played for a while. It suddenly occurred to us that George never actually suggested we play, and that Errol took the initiative whether we played at our place or theirs. So, as an experiment we decided to wait for George to invite us to play. Well we very much regretted this later, for although George often remarked that it was a while since we had played, Errol refrained from saying as usual, 'What about a game of cards?', or, 'Are you free tonight?' What started out as a bit of fun believing that George would actually ask us, did not end that way. Then I wondered had they ever really wanted to play. By then it was too late to rectify and unfortunately the end of our card nights. We remained friends but lost touch when they moved to the Lakeshore. George started playing tennis elsewhere and Dot was busy with family living in that area.

The wonderful thing is that we caught up with them forty years later when in Sydney, and found that they had moved to Australia years before. When we met again they were living on the Central Coast just an hour's drive north of us. We have seen them regularly and picked up our friendship where we left off. Sadly, George died shortly before last Christmas (2002).

The year before my arrival Errol had made contact with Geoff Shannon, who was the Vice-Consul at the Australian Consulate and living in New York. Geoff was from South Australia and friend of Errol's brother Ivor. Following this contact, Geoff and Errol decided to holiday together, and toured the Eastern Seaboard from Maine to New York in Errol's car. Geoff, like so many New Yorkers living in Manhattan did not own a car, so he took a train to Burlington where they arranged to meet. When Errol asked how he would recognise him, Geoff replied that it would not be a problem as he was six feet nine! The two obviously got on well. After our marriage, Geoff generously said that whenever we wished to take holidays, he would arrange to take his and we could stay in his apartment. We could not believe such generosity and took advantage of his offer the following year. We drove in Errol's car through some of the most beautiful country in the US, a trip we were to repeat many times in the future and never tired of.

Thirty years later when we drove from New York to Montreal, the new highway had bypassed all the delightful towns, lakes and beauty spots we loved so much. We missed the views of Lake George and made a point of leaving the highway in order to visit one town we had always enjoyed beside Lake Champlain. To our horror, this beautiful town had lost all of its former character, now replaced by gaudy signs and jazzy motels lining the main street, which I can only describe as honky-tonk or like a mini Las Vegas. We could not leave fast enough. If however one has the time to leave the highway, one may see many towns that have not suffered this fate. One finds the same in other countries, particularly in Europe where villages have not changed for centuries.

Our drive into Manhattan was comparatively simple and we found Geoff's apartment without difficulty, parking in a car park almost next door. Unbelievably, the building was within a street or two of the Rochester Center, the Australian Consulate and just around the corner from the United Nations. It could not have been more central, and was very convenient for us as we spent all our time out doing the town. The tiny apartment comprised of a living room with a double bed that pulled out from the wall, and a small kitchen at one end and a bathroom. The most amazing thing, even in 1953, was that during the day we could park outside on the street, though at night we put the car in the car park for security. The apartment was right in the centre of Manhattan and, from memory, it was on 45th Street. When we could, we walked, taking public transport only to go further afield. We covered the city sights and beyond: Broadway, Times Square, Hyde Park, the zoo, Fifth Avenue and its shops, Tiffanys, the Empire State building, the Guggenheim Museum and by ferry to Staten Island, around Manhattan, and to the Statue of Liberty. We took elevators and then steps right up the arm and hand holding the torch. That tour is no longer available for fear of further deterioration of the statue. We paid a visit to the Australian Consulate where we met Geoff's colleagues. They included Ron Gray, their Chief Financial Officer, who invited us to his home for a barbecue on the following Sunday. It was a friendly Aussie get-together and there we met and became instant friends with Norm and Midge Bentley. We liked and got on well with Ron and Wendy Gray too, and on subsequent visits to New York we saw them until their return to Australia. Norm Bentley was English and had met Midge shortly after the war when she was holidaying in England. After their marriage, they went to New York to live. They had no children, though their widowed mothers became best friends and lived together for many years - until Midge's mother's death. The Bentleys lived in White Plains, half an hour north of Manhattan by train, while Norm's mother, Tich, had a small apartment with her little poodle in nearby Scarborough. Tich was a lot of fun and unlike the proverbial mother-in-law. Midge could do no wrong in her eyes; the feeling was mutual. Years later, we returned over the summer holidays to Montreal and New York with our children - Trevor, Ross and Jennifer. (Jennifer had her twelfth birthday twice on the plane, as we crossed the International Dateline and celebrated with a cake on each day.) We spent Christmas and a wonderful week with the Bentleys (Norm is Trevor's godfather), and visited Tich. When Jennifer saw the bejewelled poodle with his sparkling collar, her eyes opened wide as she asked, 'Are they real diamonds?' to which Tich replied, 'Is there anything else?'

Our first visit to New York in 1954 was not our last, for we returned often, always staying with Norm and Midge. We have cherished memories of the laughter and happy times spent in their company. Throughout our years in Montreal, they too visited us on their way to the Laurentian Mountains for skiing, and on occasions at Christmas or New Year, we accompanied them. At Easter 1955, we met them again with Geoff Shannon in Jay Peak, Vermont, where they skied. Meanwhile we drove and walked around the villages and countryside so unique to Vermont, where every season is breathtakingly beautiful. At that time of year, the mountains still have their mantle of snow, and while the ground has a covering the thaw is setting in; ice is slowly melting in streams, as is the snow on logs and trees. Twigs dripping with icicles are sheer magic, and branches, bare and wet dark brown, are patterned with the remaining snow. In the streams, the water trickles around stones crowned with the last snow and rushes over little waterfalls. The thaw presents a different picture on the roads where all becomes dirty slush from the speeding cars, which leave a trail in their wake as they toss the slush aside onto the banks of once sparkling white snow. Then, suddenly, as days become warmer all comes alive and within a week bare trees burst into leaf, magnolias flower, and crocuses pop up in the damp soil. In Montreal spring always came with such suddenness in mid-April that we never ceased to be amazed.

I met Gwen Winnicki through a friend of Fuff's, who was working in Montreal. Gwen, an Australian from Bowen, Queensland, was married to a Latvian whom she had met in London. Gwen worked for a solicitor also on Greene Avenue and she often came into the bank. As they lived nearby, we asked them to dinner and very soon became good friends. When they arrived for that first dinner, we were surprised to see Ludick at six feet seven, towering over Gwen's tiny five feet two figure. We saw a lot of them, especially Gwen, as Lu was very jealous and she kept leaving him for the shelter of our home. Wherever she was, he hunted her down, and she being a devout Catholic was loathe to leave him permanently. She valiantly accompanied him to Newfoundland when he was transferred for a year as a mining engineer. Eventually the marriage was annulled, and after we left Montreal, Gwen went to Paris to improve her French at the Sorbonne and onto Geneva where she worked for the United Nations. There she met and married James Halsey, a New Yorker who was also extremely tall. James was the son of Fleet Admiral 'Bull' Halsey of WWII fame, well known for coining the naval motto, 'Hit harder, hit fast, hit often', and his motivational posters with the 'Kill Japs!!! Kill Japs!!! Kill more Japs!!!' On returning to New York, they moved into their apartment in the exclusive Sutton Place on Manhattan Island, very central and convenient both to James' workplace and to the United Nations where Gwen worked. Gwen told us that walking to and from work at odd hours and around Manhattan at night never bothered her, and because New Yorkers were recognised as such, they were never worried about being attacked as tourists might be. She said that a fellow Australian, who had lived for years on the other, less desirable side of Manhattan, felt the same way. On trips from Australia to New York, we have visited them when staying with the Bentleys. Trevor has visited and stayed with them and they all get on very well. Gwen and James have no children, and she has a soft spot for Trevor as she saw a lot of him when a baby. Had Gwen not been of the Catholic faith (most of our close friends were), we would have asked her to be his godmother. Two years ago, both now retired they moved to the house they had built in Bridgehampton, Long Island, where James grew up. We have all kept in touch, sent letters at Christmas and met in Sydney on their visits to Australia.

A most lovely apartment - Monkland Avenue

Three years after our marriage we moved to a newly built apartment building on 5900 Monkland Avenue, Notre Dame de Grace. Our apartment on the top floor had a balcony that overlooked the Monkland tennis courts, and beyond to Loyola College grounds with a fine view of the Catholic Church steeple. Errol lost no time in telling Ed McAsey that the steeple might bring us closer to the faith and was the reason we were attracted to the apartment! Ed as usual took it all in good humour. Our new home was sunny and open with large windows. The front door opened in to a small entrance and a long L-shaped passage. The shorter passage had a bathroom on the right and then led into the kitchen. The longer passage had a second bedroom or study off to the right and at the end opened into a larger area and the main bedroom and living room with a large balcony. Both these rooms had expansive views, as did the kitchen. The apartment being new was modern and very roomy like a home. We had the fun of furnishing, buying all new furniture except for Errol's maple bedroom suite. We bought new curtains to cover the wall-to-wall windows in the living room, and to colour coordinate with the new lounge suite. We bought a carpet runner for the passage and our piece de resistance was a pair of magnificent Indian carpets for the living and our bedroom. I believe our apartment was the envy of all our friends, all of whom lived in apartments with the exception of Ed and Inez and a few living further out on the Lakeshore. Unfortunately, we did not own the apartment; nor did anyone we knew, as all apartment buildings were owned by consortia. Over the eight or nine year period when we paid exorbitant rent, we could have bought several homes, but we always believed that our stay in Canada would be short term. One casual job I had after arriving was in a new high-rise block on Cote St Luc, handing out brochures and letting the apartments.

When we moved to Monkland Avenue it was further to the bank, and although it took no more than fifteen minutes by streetcar, I decided to resign. I was offered a job by Bill Manners, whom I knew as a non-playing member of the tennis club. Bill was a Director of United Amusement, the company that owned all the cinemas in Toronto, and many in Montreal. What appealed most was that their offices were immediately opposite our apartment. There were six of us in the general office, and three directors and two staff in the executive offices. I was employed as a bookkeeper and relief telephonist, and soon realised my good fortune in having such friendly and cooperative fellow workmates. Therefore, it was a happy place and no one was over-worked. Sometimes the Chairman, Mr Lester, bought cakes to have with our coffee, and occasionally he took us out to lunch at Ruby

Foos Chinese Restaurant, the best restaurant on the island. Freshly brewed coffee, always made by Genny Copeman, was a ritual each morning and afternoon. Genny, a little older than me, was a member of the tennis club and after a while, we played during the lunch hour. I had not known Genny well before nor had I particularly liked her, for she and her friends were very loud and boisterous. They sat in a group apart from the rest of us and as long time members, they acted as though they owned the club - or so it seemed. While working with Genny I realised what a kind person she was, and from then on, we became very close friends. Genny later confessed to me that she was actually very shy, and that her loud confident manner was a cover-up. I have since learned how wrong first impressions can be and that the face people present to the world can cover up some insecurity. None of our children ever prejudges and I try to follow their example.

Around the time of our moving and after Selby's death, Errol was very disillusioned with his appointment and responsibilities at The Foundation Company. He applied for the position of Assistant Treasurer at the Canadian Car and Foundry, which was a subsidiary of the British Hawker Siddley Group and a convenient ten-minute drive from home.

We made new friends through the tennis club. Malcolm (a Scot) and Wendy (English) Ferrier newly arrived in Canada became good friends with whom we played tennis, bridge and spent weekends in The Laurentians in the snow. Later they moved to Chalk River, near Ottawa, where Malcolm an industrial chemist worked as technical librarian at the nuclear reactor plant. Wendy was also a chemist but as they soon started a family, she did not work outside the home. One Christmas we visited them and their small sons, Neil and Fergus, who were to be the first of four, when Trevor was eight months old and I was four months pregnant with Ross. We still keep in touch at Christmas, and many years later after they had moved to San Diego, we stayed with them. On their travels our children too have visited them, the boys in San Diego and Jennifer when they lived on Vancouver Island.

Our closest Canadian friends, Bunny and John Scholes, were our first neighbours in the Monkland apartment - our two doors side by side. A week or so before they moved out, Errol met Bunny who opened their door believing that it was John. Bunny invited us for a drink and then they asked if we would like to see their new home, just completed in the new suburb of Preville, across the Jacques Cartier Bridge on the other side of the St Lawrence River. There on developed a beautiful friendship and an exchange of visits and dinners. Both Bunny and I regarded cooking as an art to be enjoyed in the making, as well as in the eating. Just before we returned to Australia they were transferred to Toronto, but we have kept in touch ever since. They have stayed with us in Sydney, and we with them once in Toronto - as too have our boys.

Also, as a family on our return visit in 1974, we stayed over the New Year with them and their family at their 'shack', which proved to be a four-storey chalet in Vermont. As with many homes in that part of the world, the chalet had a huge basement area with rumpus and games room, an extra bedroom, bathroom, storage, laundry, and drying area - Canadians rarely hang clothes outside. There was a kitchen and huge living room on the first floor, and four bedrooms with balconies and bathrooms on the top floors. Just a small weekender! We had a wonderful time in the snow, tobogganing and walking while the Scholes skied. Though the temperature was below zero, it was so warm with the white snow reflecting the sun's rays. In fact, when Jennifer and I were out walking, we stripped down to our blouses, as we got so hot. The Scholes were generous hosts taking us out and entertaining neighbours. Bunny coped amazingly well feeding ten of us magnificent meals including cooking a turkey. All seemed effortless, not to mention the preparation required beforehand. In spite of their busy lifestyle, she has never had any domestic help in any of their homes. Incidentally, their four-storey terrace in Toronto, a stone's throw from the centre of the city, also had five bedrooms and four bathrooms. Recently they moved to Ottawa to be close to their daughter and five grandchildren, and are living almost next door to Government House and the Royal

Ottawa Golf Club. Despite their obvious wealth, they are both completely down to earth.

The family trip was organised to show our boys where they were born. After our stay with the Bentleys, we took the train from New York to Montreal where John picked us up and then after Vermont returned us to very good friends Jean and Eric Glencross in Lachine. (Jean had worked at The Foundation Company.) We showed the children St Matthias Church, where we were married and where they were christened, 5900 Monkland, and all our favourite places. We introduced them to our Montreal friends, whom they have since visited on their own. Ethel and Bryant Murphy threw a party with our tennis club friends, and we took a drive to the Laurentians to Parkers Lodge, a favourite weekend haunt over our years in Montreal. It was owned by Johnnie Parker, a friend from the tennis club, who also worked with me at United Amusement. This trip initially was planned for eight weeks in Canada and the US, but as Errol was required in London on business, we flew from Montreal to England for two weeks. From there, we took advantage of an inexpensive all-inclusive package deal for a week in Malaga, a coastal resort in southern Spain. What an experience that was for us all, in a luxurious unit, Spanish cuisine, and a week of touring around in our little hire car to Ronda and Granada. A highlight too was taking the ferry from Gibraltar for a day tour in colourful Tangiers, a memorable day and another story.

While we were in London, we had dinner with the Financial Director of British Tioxide, Peter Haworth, and his wife Betty; and then they took the whole family to a stage performance of Billy, in which Michael Crawford played the lead. By the interval I felt unwell, with severe midriff body pains and the theatre managers took me with Errol to a sick room. They thought I had had a heart attack and called an ambulance. Errol and I were raced away to a hospital near Buckingham Palace, leaving the Haworths to take the children back to our flat after the show. At the hospital, the doctors eventually concluded that my problem was a severe gastric upset, probably from our pre-show dinner - much to everyone's relief. I never did get to see Michael

Crawford in the flesh! All I could think of while being rushed through the streets of London was how much the children would have enjoyed the ride, with siren screaming and all traffic giving way!

I return now to Montreal, and the time of our first meeting with the Scholes. After they left we determined that we would introduce ourselves to any new tenants, which we did, and so developed another wonderful friendship with Lorne and Doreen Hewson. One of the nicest couples we have ever met. Doreen did not work, and as we did, she insisted we go to them for supper (dinner) every Thursday night, and of course, we reciprocated but not as often. One funny thing I always remember about Lorne is that he would get up an hour early each morning, in order to lie in the bath and read before work. This always amused us. We did many things together, drives and picnics, and as they loved camping and fishing, they invited us to go away for a weekend. They took us to a beautiful spot beside a river, where we set up camp, fished, and then ate in the glow of a big fire before settling down for an early night. I was bitten so badly by mosquitoes that I had an allergic reaction, so extreme that one hand swelled to twice its size. We were forced to return home to seek medical attention. Canadian mosquitoes are indeed big and nasty, and put an end to any thoughts of further camping trips. A more enjoyable weekend was spent with the Hewsons as the guests of Ed and Marie Harvey, who also lived in our building with their adorable four-year-old daughter. The Harveys owned a chalet at a remote lake in Ontario, where we spent our time boating and learning to water ski. Almost at the stage of some expertise, I found myself entangled in the rope and with a sprained ankle, thus ending a brilliant water skiing career. No mosquitoes or even marauding bears in that idyllic place, only squirrels and friendly little chipmunks scampering about. We were fascinated by these little creatures busily running around, up and down trees, and over grass in city parks collecting their winter supplies of nuts or with luck a free hand out. They were very tame and if encouraged would happily run up arms and perch on one's head or shoulders. Errol has many photographs of them doing just this with me.

The Harveys moved away, and later the Hewsons to Ottawa though they returned and lived in Preville just before our return to Australia - by which time they and we too, had two sons. When we went as a family with our teenagers, we were so happy to see them once more. The children had much fun tobogganing and building a snowman, and I have vivid memories of Jennifer, a lone little figure outside for many hours in the dark, busily perfecting our snowman. We were so sad to learn that Doreen died from cancer when still in her late forties. She really was one of the beautiful people of this world. We kept in touch with Lorne, and he and his new wife were pleased to have Trevor and Ross stay with them in North Vancouver. In the last few years, Lorne suffered from dementia and late in the 2001, we received an email saying he had died. Dear Lorne was such a lovely happy fellow as our boys discovered on their visit. Strangely, I can still see his and Doreen's faces clearly, more so than our other old friends.

The four years we lived in that apartment were perfect, for we did so many exciting and interesting things. Among our many weekends were regular trips to Johnnie Parker's Lodge on the shores of Lake Paquin in the Laurentians - about an hour's drive north of Montreal. Six or so couples from the tennis club would take over the lodge for a weekend of fun and hilarity. It was a place for all seasons with ski slopes and a golf club nearby, and fishing, boating and swimming at the front of the grounds. As Johnnie had regular visitors from further afield, Ontario, the US, and even from overseas, we avoided the high seasons so we could have the place to ourselves. Besides, it ensured that Johnnie always had a full house. Owing to its intimacy, the lodge was very popular, and being run by the owners added that personal touch. Helen ran the kitchen producing fabulous home-cooked meals, always with delicious corn bread baked on the premises. Guests sat at one long table for all meals, which encouraged conversation and an ambience that allowed all guests to become acquainted. As well as outdoor pursuits, we played bridge, table tennis, and spent much time eating and drinking with great bonhomie. Suffice to say these were happy days in the company of friends. Johnnie organised twice-yearly golfing weekends for the 'boys', to which Errol invited John Scholes and Eric Glencross, who continued to attend long after our departure.

Jack Vicars, a social member of the club, invited us to Toronto to stay with his parents. We visited twice and became very good friends with Mr and Mrs Vicars and his sister Mary. They welcomed us and were very kind, treating us like family. Later when Jack became engaged to an Italian girl, his parents were very unhappy. Especially his mother, as Gisele was a Catholic and they devout Protestants. Despite this, Jack and Gisele were married in the Catholic Cathedral in the old French quarter of East Montreal. We attended the ceremony and sat with the Vicars family, where dear Mrs Vicars expressed her dismay and whispered to me, 'I never thought I would see this day.' I often wondered if she ever accepted Gisele as the marriage has lasted very happily to this day. Gisele is a very smart businesswoman and spurred Jack on in his business, and helped with financial decisions. In my opinion, she is the power behind the marriage. Errol taught Gisele to play bridge, and now she and Jack have earned their Masters status playing in the big competitions. When last we met they were living in a mansion, which Gisele bought on a whim and sold at a very handsome profit. Their three children have successful careers, all of which proves that parents should trust their children's judgement when choosing mates. In retirement Jack has a good and happy life as does Gisele, and they want for nothing.

We had been living in the new apartment for about a year when Auntie Kath wrote to tell me that Walter Fotheringham and his new bride Ann (nee Sheidow) were coming from Adelaide to Montreal for a period, and asked would we meet them. Of course we were delighted when they contacted us on arrival. They had come to Canada with two other newly married young couples, Airlie and Barry Barham-Black, and Dymphna and John Laurie. The men were good friends from St Peter's College, were all engineers, and had come to Montreal for experience. Ann was an outstanding tennis player and may even have been a member of the Australian Federation Cup team. She joined our tennis club where she outshone all other women, and no doubt most of the men. To this day she plays a strong game, and she and her partner are the current titleholders of the women's doubles over sixty-five world championship. For some years, she partnered Judy Dalton at Kooyong in Melbourne. Although they were younger, we got on well with all three couples, and invited them to spend their first Christmas with us. Thereafter we entertained each other and had a weekend visit to Quebec City, which was a lot of fun in the company of fellow Aussies. We saw more of Ann and Wally because of our tennis interest, and several times we all went to Lake Memphremagog, near Granby, to view the fall colours. What still amazes me is the number of holidays we had in our years in Canada, as I believe annual leave was only of two weeks duration. Apart from our honeymoon, we spent the following vacation in New York in Geoff's apartment. The next year we drove to NY and stayed with Midge and Norm Bentley before flying on to Florida, where we stayed at the Fontainbleu right on Miami Beach. What an eye-opener it was to see all the high-rise resort hotels lining the beach. All had cabarets and entertainment for the price of a drink, and though expensive, the experience was worth it. The Eden Roc was next door and the most luxurious. As it was off-season, we had a package deal and prices were generally low. We toured the Everglades, a crocodile reserve, an Indian reserve, and cruised the canals viewing the holiday homes of the rich and famous. As well, we swam in the pool and lazed about on lounge chairs, as one does at resorts all over the world now. None, however, is more luxurious than those at Miami Beach in the mid-fifties. Finally, we made our first (and my last) visit to a strip club – an anticlimax for both of us!

One of the nicest holidays was spent in the then quiet little backwater of Rockport on Cape Anne, just north of the historic port of Gloucester where the Pilgrims landed. We took Marg Godwin with us, and all stayed at a Cape Cod guesthouse. Breakfast was provided and we ate all other meals at Peg Legs right on the beachfront. For years we made comparisons with the lobster and huge gourmet meals served at this restaurant. There were many firsts for us. One thing I remember and have since made is a pickle from watermelon rind. We swam at the beach, but mostly visited the quaint little studios of artists along the long jetty that leads to the breakwater. Half way along there was an old wooden building, named Motif No 1, which was reputed to be the most painted subject in all of the US. We did buy a painting, not of Motif No 1, but of the countryside in the fall. We still have it in its original rustic frame. We toured the surrounding coastline and formed the opinion that Cape Anne was much more appealing than the better known Cape Cod further south.

On the Bentleys' advice we decided to visit Prince Edward Island, the home of Anne of Green Gables fame. We drove through New Hampshire to St Johns, New Brunswick, where we took a ferry to the island. A peaceful little place, we spent eight days playing golf, walking around the island, lazing on the beach, and relaxing with other guests. We viewed Green Gables, which was exactly as described in the book. My Japanese teacher and good friend, Humiko, recently told me that her Japanese mother had just realised her lifelong dream, which was to visit Green Gables before she died. The fact that not only were these books read by Japanese children fifty years ago, but that they should be of such significance came as a great surprise to me.

For us it was a relaxing holiday, though somewhat spoilt for me as I was not well. Although I was two months pregnant, that was not the cause, I was suffering from a somewhat more delicate condition. Again by ferry we returned via Halifax, Nova Scotia, which was a world apart and moved at a slower pace than the Canada we knew - like Tasmania is to mainland Australia. Peggy's Cove, shrouded in mist was a photographer's delight.

For eight years apart from holidays and touring around endeavouring to see as much as possible of this beautiful country, every hour was occupied with work, tennis, bridge and our separate hobbies. Errol always a keen photographer had bought all equipment necessary for doing his own developing and printing. In our first apartment, he set up his own dark room in the basement, where all occupants were allotted an area for storage. Somehow, he had managed to get an extra space. Here he spent night after night patiently developing, printing and enlarging, transforming film into black and white artistic creations. At Monkland Avenue, he did not have this facility, but continued with his photography. To this day, we have a wonderful pictorial record of our lives, of our children growing up and our numerous overseas trips. Wherever we can, we have tried to travel independent of groups, enabling us to visit out of the way places.

In more exotic countries like India, Egypt and Japan, Errol has captured scenes which not only bring back memories of places but those unusual experiences, some good and some not so good, which turn a holiday into an adventure. These photographs have genuinely fascinated many of our friends, by bringing alive the colour and people of these countries.

Starting a family

In 1958, Errol found a new subject for his camera when our first baby was born on the 18th April. During my pregnancy, I was determined to have the perfect baby, and followed every rule in the book. That meant a nutritious diet with plenty of fibre, including whole-grain bread, salads and skim milk, and strictly no fatty foods, cakes, pastries or cream. I also cut out salt and supplemented my diet with vitamins. After a few months, my obstetrician Dr Harry Oxorn was surprised that I had put on so little weight. When I told him my diet, he was pleased, but added that no one had ever taken his advice so seriously. At the end of nine months, I had only put on eighteen pounds (8.1 kg) and the day after giving birth was under my pre-pregnancy weight. In fact, all the nutrition of my strict diet had gone to my healthy baby of eight pounds six ounces. I had attended pre-natal exercise and breathing classes, with the intention of having a natural birth as recommended by Dr Oxorn. By keeping very active, I was able to continue working until six weeks before the birth, when I was asked the reason for my leaving. Only then did I start wearing maternity clothes, the design of which I had not seen before, or since in Australia. A two-piece outfit of a slim skirt with a hole cut out over the stomach area, which allowed for the bulge without affecting the hang of the skirt, and a loose smock over the top. Besides being most attractive and very comfortable, they effectively helped disguise the otherwise obvious bulge. I indulged myself with three bought outfits, including a pair of slacks with stretch material replacing the hole, and I made a smock with pleated front to go with the slacks. These outfits were worn for all my following pregnancies and always much admired. I have them still and as all are like new and quite fashionable, I have been hoping that our daughter, Jennifer, might want to use them.

For me the sheer wonder of giving birth was the most incredible and beautiful experience of my life, far beyond my imagination and any preconceived ideas. Each child was a true gift from God, and all have brought untold joy and happiness as time goes by. From the moment they were born, I marvelled at the growing process, which changed day by day - each child so different from the others. Never once has any of them disappointed me, and though far from perfect, I have felt only pride in their many achievements, big and small alike, and admiration for their humanity, integrity and Christian outlook. Now I am older, and in need, I count my blessings every day for the support they give both Errol and me, and their enduring love shown in countless ways. Apart from daily contact by phone, email, chat sessions on computer, and surprises by post, they have travelled frequently to assist in every way to make our lives easier. What is more, they all are highly intelligent with a wide range of interests and are much travelled. They are down-to-earth and non-materialistic, have a great sense of humour, and love of the environment and people - both young and old. What more can I say? Am I biased? No, I am just being honest! I cannot believe our good fortune in having such wonderful children. Of course, Errol, the love of my life has had considerable input too.

We had always planned to return to Australia before starting a family, but then fate stepped in and decided otherwise. Dr Harry Oxorn on Guy Street was recommended, and was dedicated, kind and caring, and had a good sense of humour. They say all pregnant women fall in love with their obstetrician, which I guess I did. The pregnancy did not interfere with our lifestyle except change some of my eating habits. Although we told none of our friends about the coming event, Yolan Gregor told me later that she guessed when we were playing bridge at her place, she had noticed my heavy breathing and that had I refused the dessert. She lived with her parents, Hungarian migrants, who had escaped from their homeland when she was a child. Her father was a baker with his own shop, which was renowned for its delicious pastries.

It was a straightforward pregnancy with no problems whatsoever, apart from a nagging cold and very sore throat. I turned to Dr Oxorn, who in his wisdom said he did not believe in prescribing any unnecessary drugs during pregnancy because of the many unknown side effects. He advised me to use only Vitamin C and natural products. How right he was, as 1958 was the period when thalidomide was prescribed and many malformed babies were born. All due to some simple drug thought to be harmless to pregnant women and their unborn babies!

After stopping work, I spent much time cleaning and polishing the wooden floors not covered by carpet, so much so that Errol jokingly said that I would take the vacuum to hospital. Fortnightly I went downtown to collect my twenty-two dollars unemployment benefit, to which I was entitled if I had been sacked. Most employers obligingly said that an employee was put off rather than had resigned, and as all employees paid into this fund it seemed fair enough to get some of it back. Errol fell into the category of those earning high salaries, who though they contributed, were not entitled to receive benefits. At first I was shocked, but everyone took advantage of the system, even Claire Knight, who drove down in her new Buick and fronted up to the counter in her mink coat. I decided to join the queue. I collected for over twelve months and during that time received only a fraction of what I had paid in. The policy was that one could refuse no more than three jobs offered within a certain radius of home, before the allowance would stop. Because I was last employed as a telephonist/bookkeeper, any job offered had to be in that line of work. There were very few offices in our area and I was only ever offered one job, which required a telephonist fluent in French.

On 17th April 1958, after a busy day collecting my dole and shopping I returned home. Just before dinner, I suddenly felt mild contractions, which increased as the evening progressed. We left for The Queen Victoria Hospital where Dr Oxorn soon joined us. After a long hard labour with Errol beside me, I delivered a beautiful boy around seven a.m., 18th April 1958. He was soon to be named Trevor Leslie, the latter being a family name for the first-born son. Believing that putting on little weight would ensure an easy birth and a small baby, I was in for a surprise as it was the reverse. Trevor was a big baby (eight lbs six oz) and the delivery as long and arduous as I had never imagined. I distinctly remember feeling as though I was climbing up the walls in an effort to escape the pain. As I was used to hiding my feelings I was embarrassed by the noise I had made, though I was assured it was quite normal. Afterwards when the doctor said, 'It was all worth it wasn't it?' my reply was 'Like hell it was!' and silently vowed never to go through it again! Despite this reaction, I was awestruck by the actual delivery, which I observed throughout in the big mirror set high on the wall opposite. I am glad that I was not sedated and was fully aware of the miracle of birth.

Of course within hours I was convinced that it was all worth it, and knew I would endure anything for our adorable son, and others if so blessed. He was the most perfect baby that anyone could wish for, gurgled and happy from morning until night, and within a few weeks slept through the night from eleven to six. I soon put him on demand feeding (popular at the time) as he was so contented, which meant I fed him when he awakened. He never fussed or cried for long when put down. As recommended by Dr Spock, I am sure the secret was that we put him in his crib and walked out of his room closing the door behind us. I took him for his six-week check-up to the paediatrician, Dr Richard Chamberlain, who very conveniently had his surgery right next door to our apartment building. The doctor was very thorough and at birth had given him a clean bill of health (apart from a slight heart murmur, which he later grew out of), so I was very alarmed to learn that he was three pounds under his birth weight. Weighing him before and after each feed soon proved that he was only getting half of what he should be. Despite the fact that I was on a very nutritious diet, I was not producing the milk for His Majesty. I then supplemented with cow's milk and within no time he was a chubby little baby with no change in his temperament. Our friends were surprised that we did not notice Trevor had not put on weight, but we knew no other babies with whom to make a comparison nor any other reason to worry.

Otherwise, it was thrilling to witness the day-by-day changes of a small baby. I feel to this day that mothers and fathers, who do not have the daily care of their children, are missing out on the many wonders of creation. We were determined to be present and to enjoy every moment, and I soon obtained the services of a reliable baby-minding service for my occasional outings. The wife of our janitor was also available at night if needed.

Son No. 2

Trevor was four months old and still feeding, when fate stepped in again and it was confirmed that I was pregnant. This news was quite unexpected to say the least, as we were just getting used to playing parents, enjoying our firstborn and not ready for another baby. Besides, I was seriously considering taking Trevor home to visit my parents whom I had not seen for seven years.

However as so often is the case, the unexpected proves to be the most rewarding and one would not wish otherwise. At daybreak 15th April 1959 and in the belief that labour would be quicker the second time round, we did not delay in our dash to hospital. It was early afternoon before our little second son entered this world, weighing in at nine pounds three ounces! We named him Ross Andrew, and though I preferred Andrew Ross, it was just as well I did not get my way, as two years later we had two little Andrews as neighbours, Andrew Neville and Andrew Gill. Our children saw more of the latter and when he was around four, Ross started referring to himself as Ross

Andrew Gill Burdon! What a different temperament Ross had right from birth. He was not as easy from the beginning, only because the poor little fellow could not digest cow's milk, which I used to supplement my inadequate supply. He brought up every meal and cried a lot, until the paediatrician put him on soymilk, which solved the problem. To this day he does not like cow's milk, no matter how disguised with flavouring. When young he used to pour milk on his cereal and then pour it off after eating the cereal. One day when Errol saw him and accused him of wasting milk, being stubborn and with a mind of his own, he refused to use milk. He replaced it with apple juice, which to this day, forty-three years on, he still does. He, like Trevor, put on weight and was much happier on the soymilk. Both boys were very active, healthy, and never had a cold despite the weather. In his first winter, Trevor had a bout of croup, which is a nightmare for any parent to watch over and to give inhalations in a steaming bathroom to a baby gasping for breath. The doctor advised that should Trevor have extreme difficulty breathing, to shove his head out the window because the cold air would force him to catch his breath. Further to our amazement, he also advised that we put Trevor back in his cot just as he was, without a sheet or any covering over him. The room was heated to 70 °Fahrenheit, sufficient for a baby while encouraging his body to heat naturally. So, this was how both boys slept from then on without any problems. The only worry we had with Ross, was when at a few weeks old he came out in a strange spotty rash on his upper body. Of great concern to his doctor, I recall the fear I had in the hospital when cuddling this tiny baby. All tests were clear and after some treatment, the rash went away.

Ross was an amazing baby and even though it seems impossible, he actually turned himself over at eight days old, a feat not normally achieved for some weeks or months. As with Trevor, I bathed him in a baby bath and dried him on the kitchen table. I turned my back for a second (something considered quite safe with a baby that age), and when I turned around, he was laying the opposite way on his stomach! We furnished their room with two matching cots with sides that could be lowered, as the child grew older, and a matching chest of drawers. We also bought attachable rails, which extended the sides another couple of feet to prevent them falling out if attempting to climb. One day we entered their room to find Ross balancing on top of the extension rail, and Trevor a year older, just standing in his cot looking on. While Trevor was very advanced but sensibly cautious, Ross was much more adventurous and often led the way. As a consequence, we tended to forget that Ross was actually a year younger, and expected him to do the same as his elder brother. When he was fifteen months, we were in a playground with the boys and turned around to see Ross at the top of a huge slide and about to slide down - which of course he did, very successfully! This risk-taking has continued throughout his life, whereas Trevor would and still does carefully contemplate the risks before making a move. As a little boy Ross was also very stubborn, a trait for which I had always blamed Errol, until Auntie Kath on observing his behaviour, remarked that he was exactly like me as a child! He grew out of this in his teens but I have many examples of such behaviour, which can now be described more accurately as an independent spirit. Trevor too is independent but in a different way. Being the eldest in the family, he took his responsibilities very seriously as a child, allowing Ross to be more carefree. Later in life Ross has become more responsible, though he still is carefree and thinks of himself as twenty-three rather than forty-three. The boys have a lot in common and can discuss any subject at great length with each other.

    The following two winters were great fun going out every day in the snow. The boys looked very cute in their red and blue snowsuits and loved tumbling and playing in the snow. I had an amazing baby carriage (pram), which converted to a stroller that could seat two back-to-back. The carriage was a Canadian design and by pressing a lever, one could raise or lower the front wheels to negotiate stairs. I coped easily with the three levels of stairs to our apartment.

    When I was pregnant with Ross, we contemplated buying a house and looked on the Lakeshore in the new suburb of Beaconsfield. We paid a five hundred dollar deposit on a split-level three-bedroom home, which had a full basement with a large rumpus room, laundry and drying area. The McAseys and Mrs Meagher came with us, and what delighted us all was the new vogue en suite bathroom. On returning to our lovely apartment, however, we decided against the move as we felt if we could manage there with one child we could probably manage with two. The apartment was convenient to all our interests, doctors, babysitter and the supermarket, whereas the house would be a slippery walk in winter months to local transport and amenities. Besides, owning a home could have delayed any return to Australia. Fortunately, we were able to retract our offer and our deposit was returned.

In the meantime, our English friends Tony and Stella Bennett had moved back to Montreal and into the next apartment. We had befriended them at the tennis club some years before Tony was transferred to Ontario. Tony was a pharmaceutical salesman and had always dropped in over the years to see me when in the neighbourhood. He was most entertaining and we had a lot in common. I was very attracted to him, as I know he was to me. When Ross was only a week old, Errol went away as planned for a golfing weekend. I was upset at being left alone to cope with my new baby and a one-year old. As Stella was still in Ontario and Tony back in Montreal, he looked after the boys and me over the weekend, taking us to visit friends, and me out dinner and to a film. I do not know what the janitor's wife, who babysat thought, but I know I have never been so close to being unfaithful as then. Had Tony not been such a good and loyal friend of Errol's, it would have happened. When the Bennetts came back to Montreal they had by then two children, Stephen and Wendy, and so we spent a lot of time in their company. After we left Montreal, we heard they split up, which did not surprise us, as Tony was so outgoing and by contrast Stella was very quiet. ~o~

Photo Pages II

A gallery can be viewed at A Quality Life, www.theburdons.com.

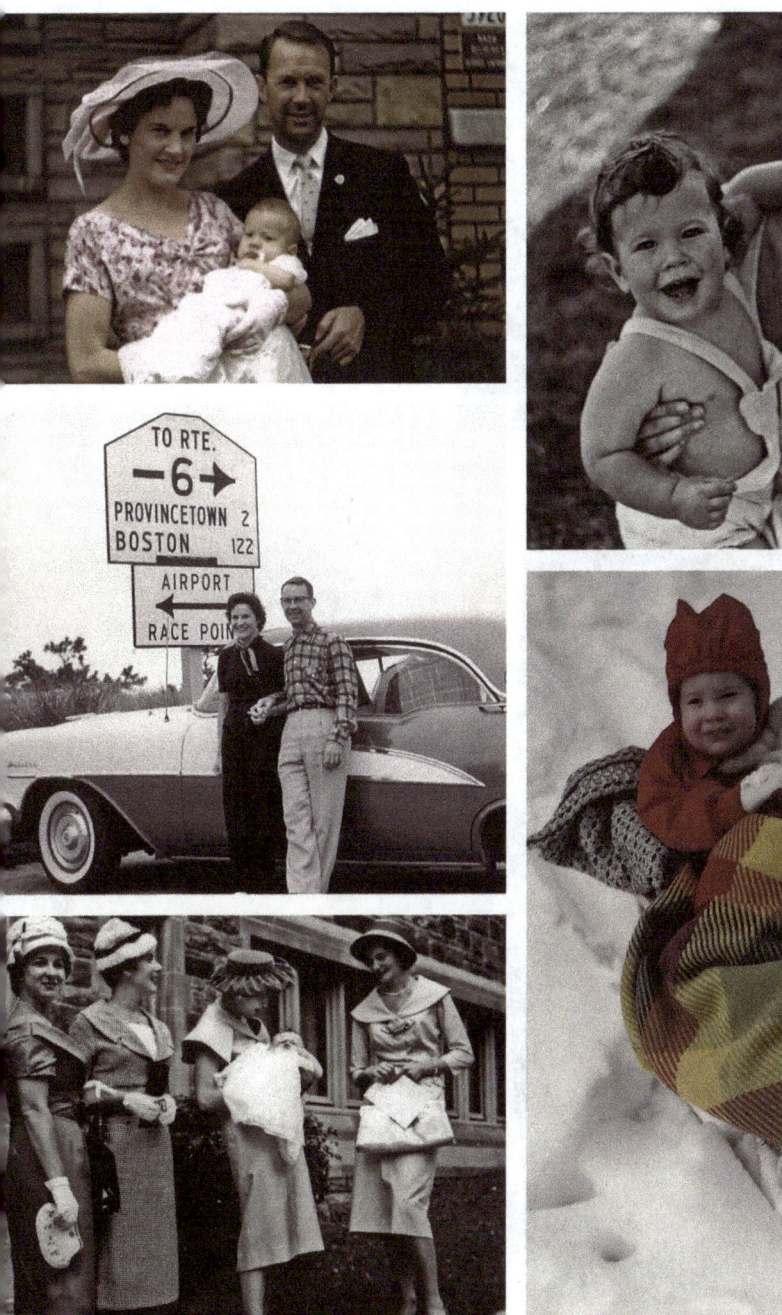

Clockwise: Trevor's christening, St Mathias, Montreal, 24 Aug 1958; Trevor & June, Monkland Tennis Club, Montreal 1959; Trevor and Ross sledding, Montreal, Xmas 1959; Ross' christening, Clare Knight, Ethel Murphy, June & Bunny Scholes, Montreal 1959; June & Errol on vacation Cape Cod 1959.

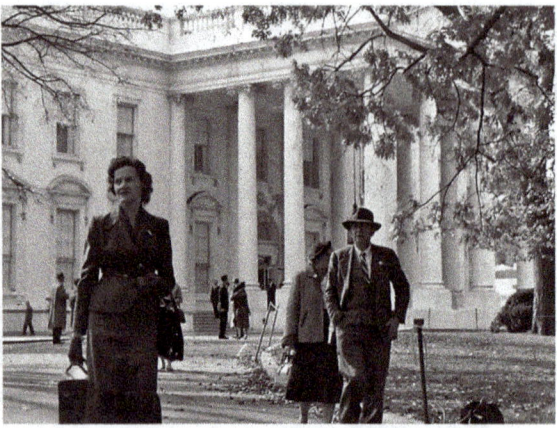
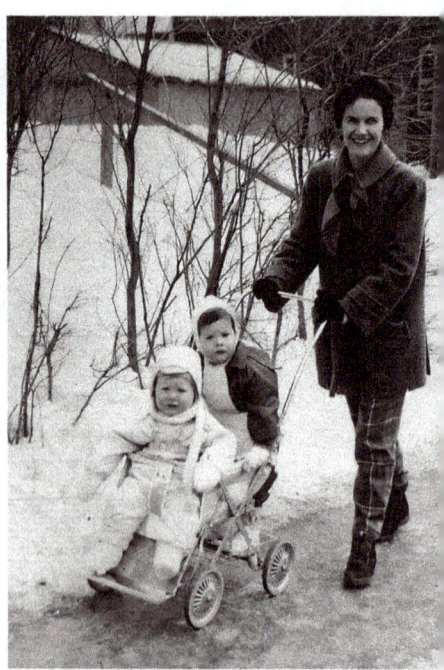
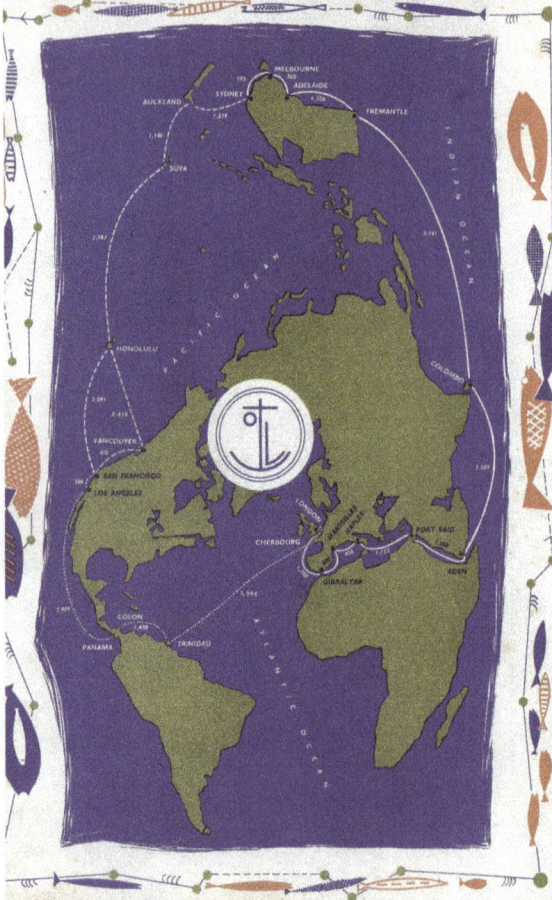
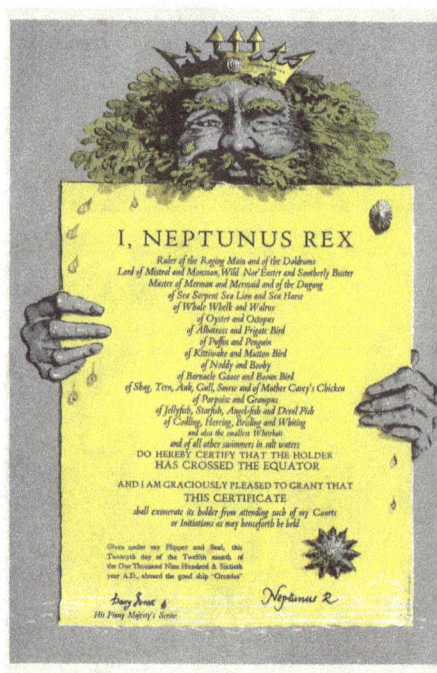

Clockwise: June at the White House, Washington, Oct 1959; Ross & Trevor in early double stroller with June, Montreal 1960; King Neptune's Certificate for crossing the Equator, 1960; SS Orcades sailing routes 1960.

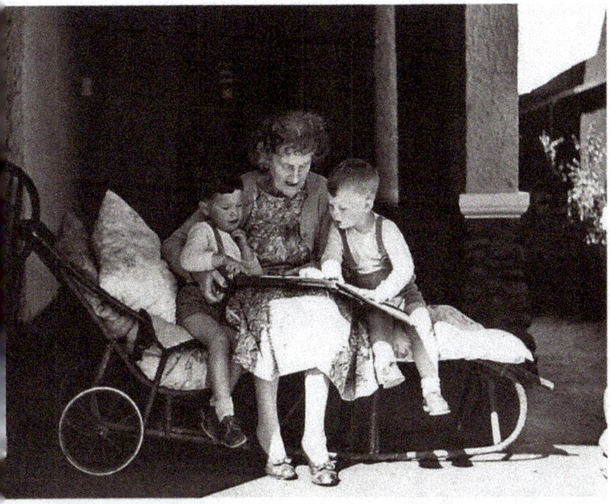

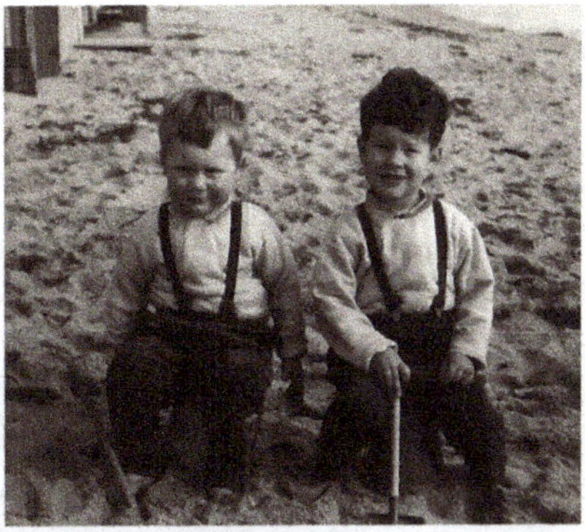

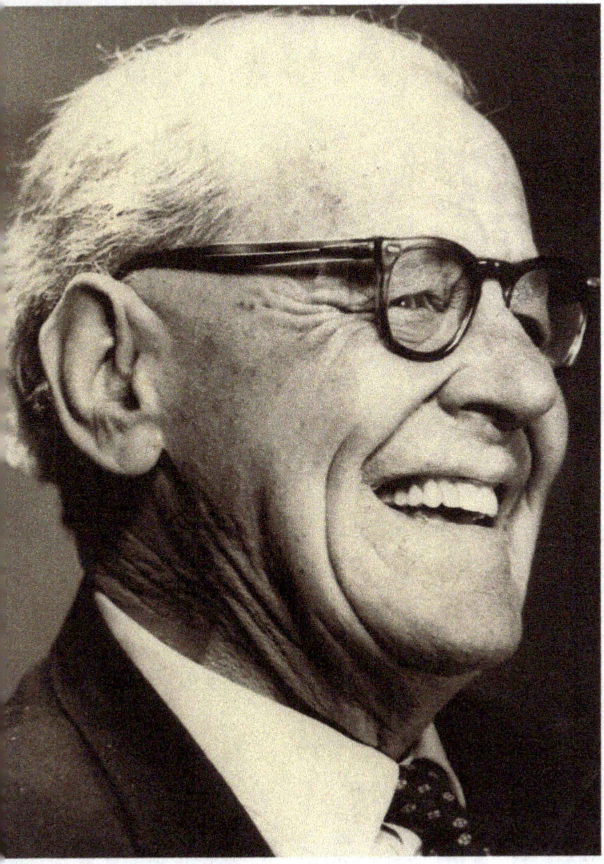

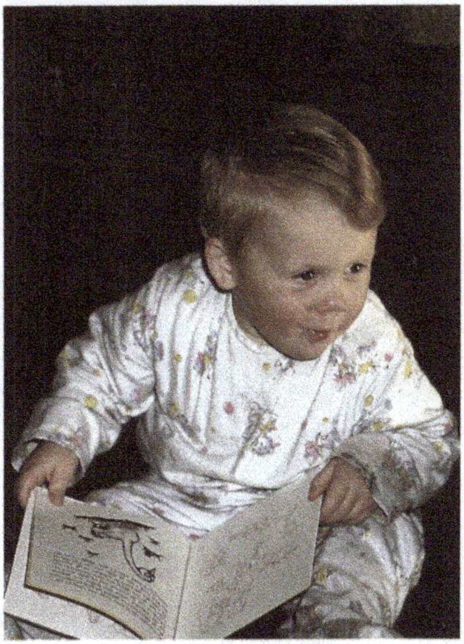

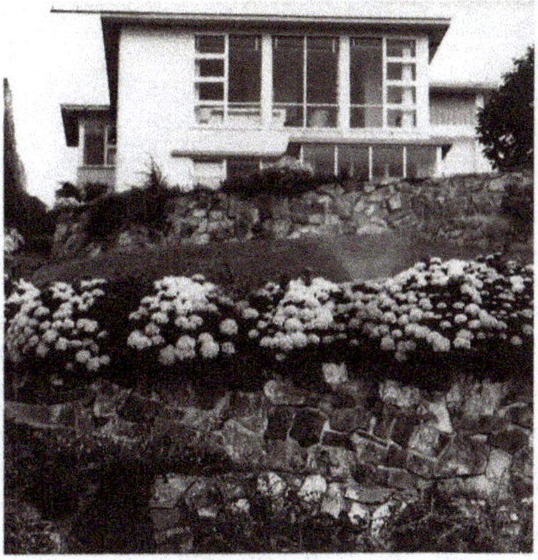

Clockwise: Aunt Kath reading to the boys, Grandfathers house, Glenelg 1962; Ross & Trevor on the beach, Melbourne 1961; Ross, Melbourne 1961; A commanding view, 25 Seaview Ave, Burnie, Tas 1962; Father Guy Herbert Dollman 1961.

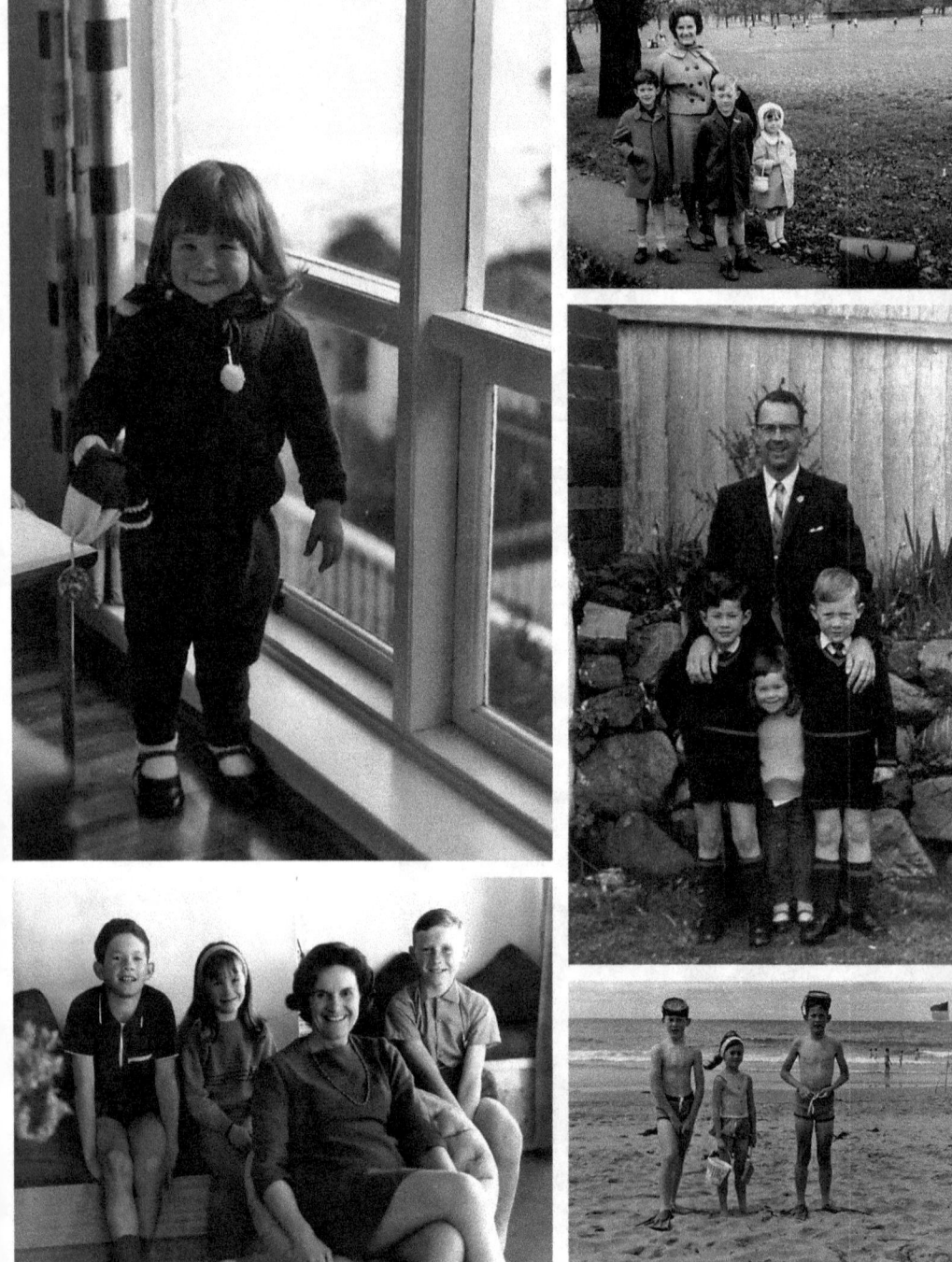

Clockwise: Jennifer in the sunroom at Seaview Ave 1964; Trevor, June, Ross & Jennifer, Adelaide c1965; Errol with brood before work, Seaview Ave c1964; Ross, Jennifer and Trevor, Boat Harbour 1967; Trevor, Jennifer, June & Ross, Seaview Ave, Burnie 1968.

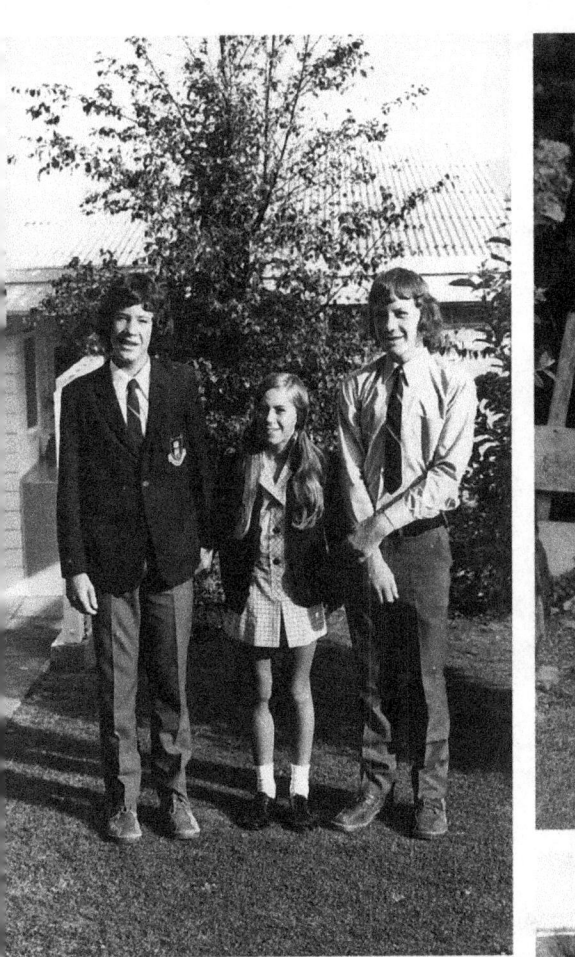
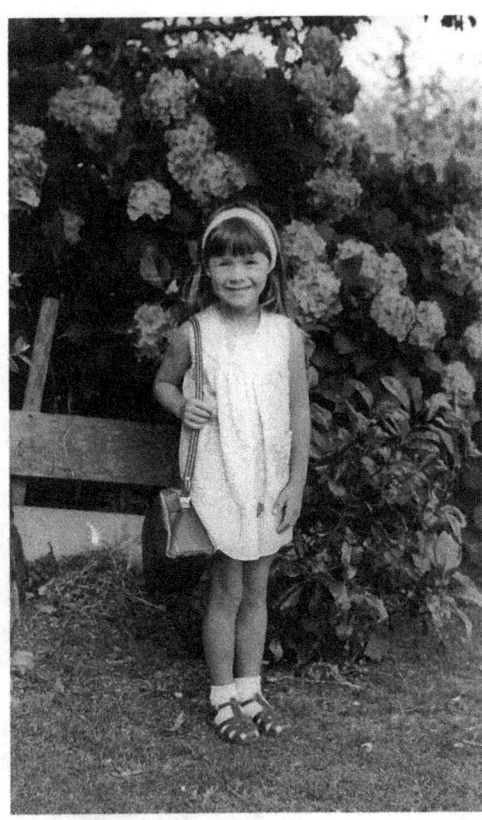
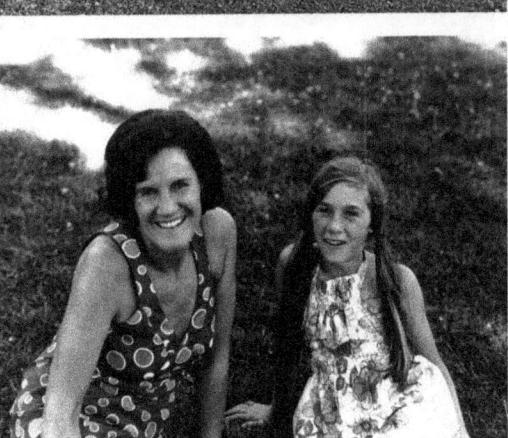
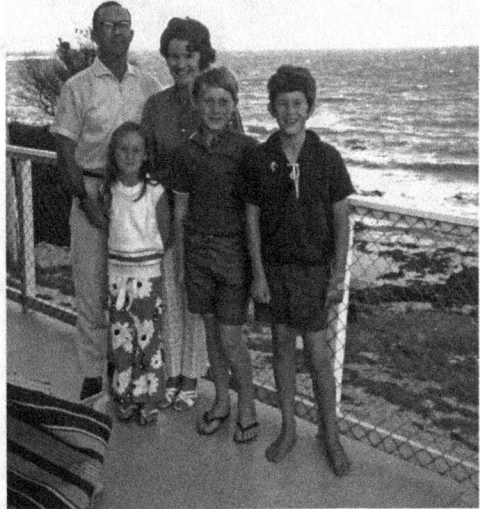

Clockwise: Before school, backyard Seaview Ave 1973; Junior Flyer Jennifer, Seaview Ave 1966; The family at Neville's shack, Boat Harbour, Tas c1969; June and Jennifer in nice dresses 1969.

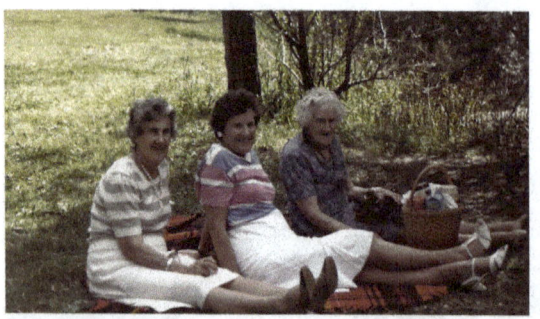
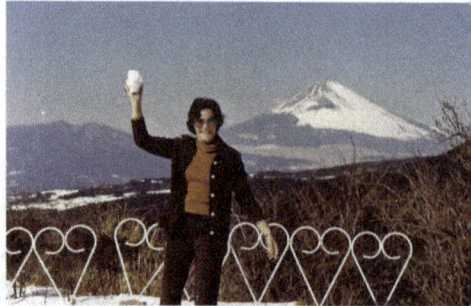
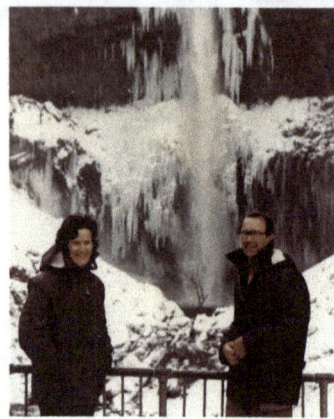
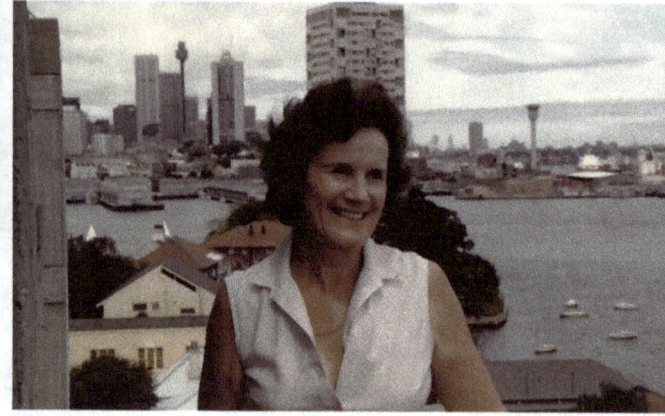

Clockwise: Fuff, June & Aunt Kath, Royal National Park, NSW, c1983; June with soft cone, Mt Fuji, Japan 1977; June hosting Japanese ladies for lunch, Finlay Rd c1984; June on the verandah of Errol's pad, Milsons Point, Sydney, Sep 1979; June & Errol at frozen waterfall, Taiwan, 1977.

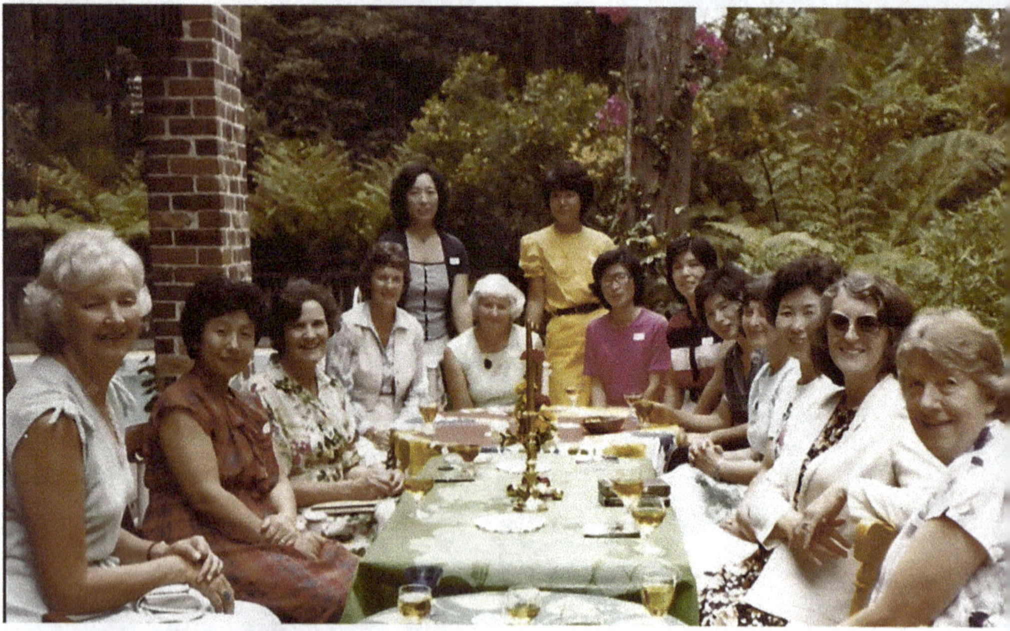

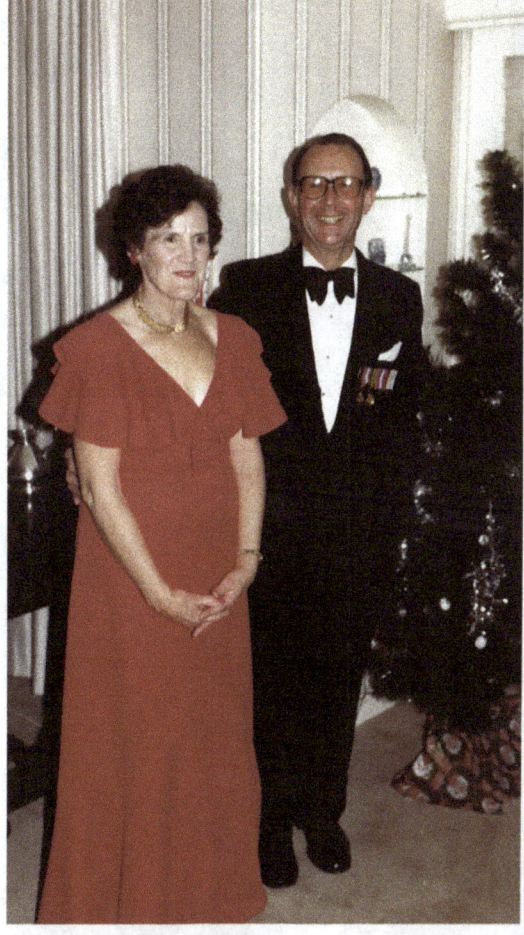

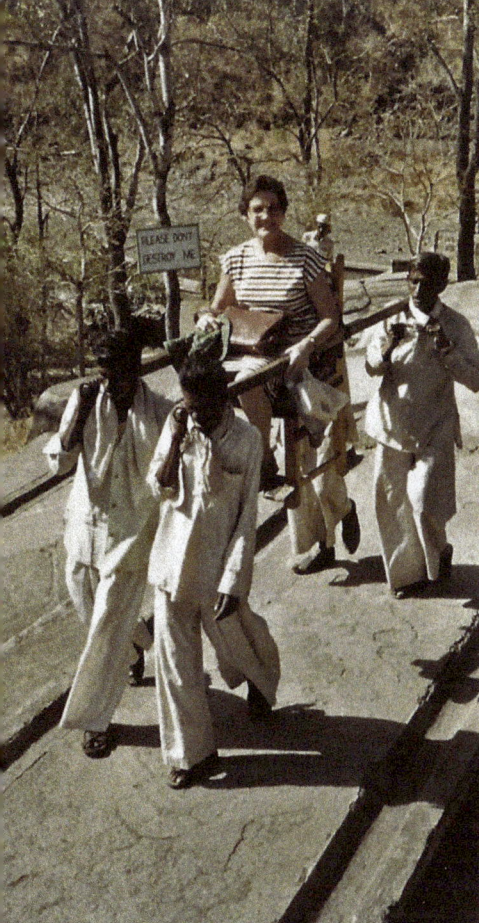

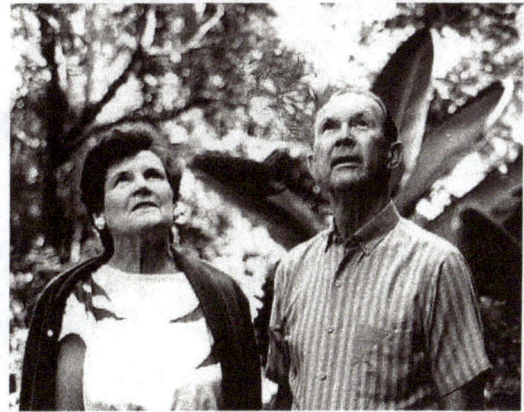

Clockwise: Elegance Evening invitation, 1984; June & Errol at McPherson's Elegance Party, Killara 1984; June & Errol, Finlay Rd, Warrawee, NSW c1985; June stretchered out in style, Aurangabad, India 1985.

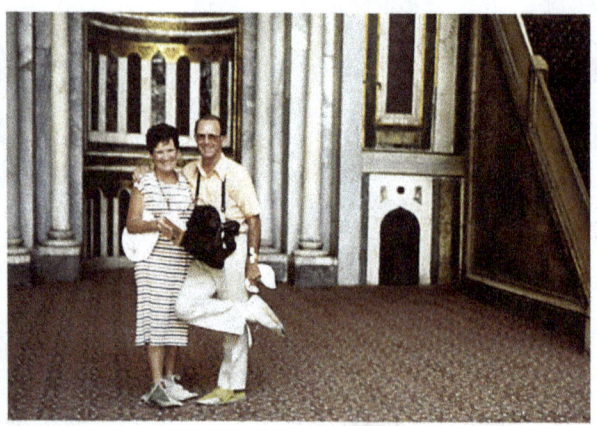
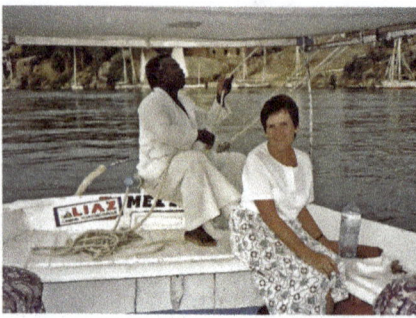
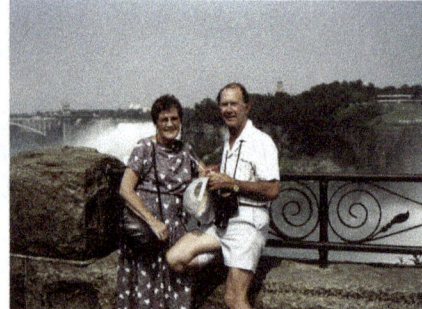
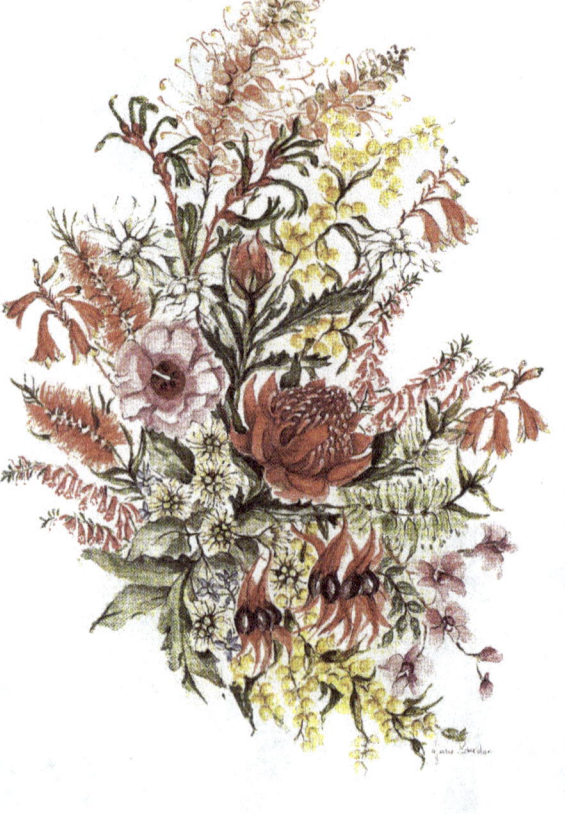
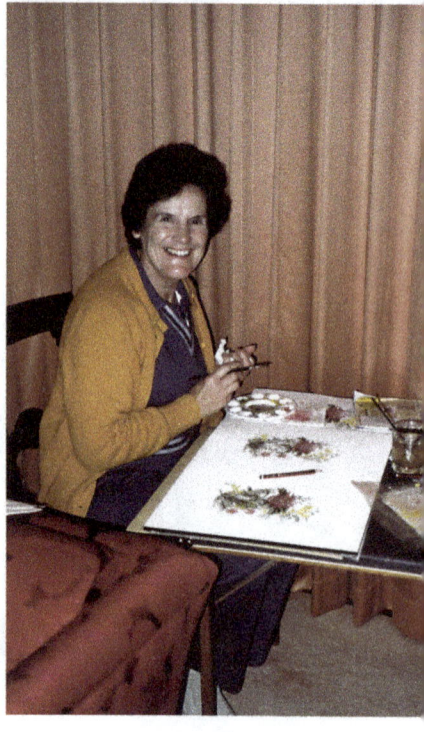

Clockwise: Adjusting footwear at a Cairo mosque 1989; June cruising the Nile, Aswan, Egypt 1989; June & Errol relive honeymoon, Niagara Falls 1989; June working on her flower sketches, Finlay Rd 1996; A popular card - #25 Floral Emblems of Australia. (See all at flowercards.com.au.)

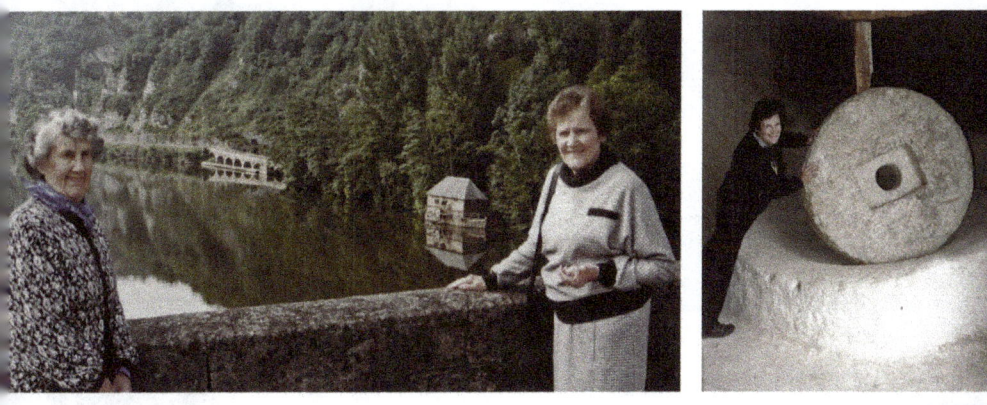
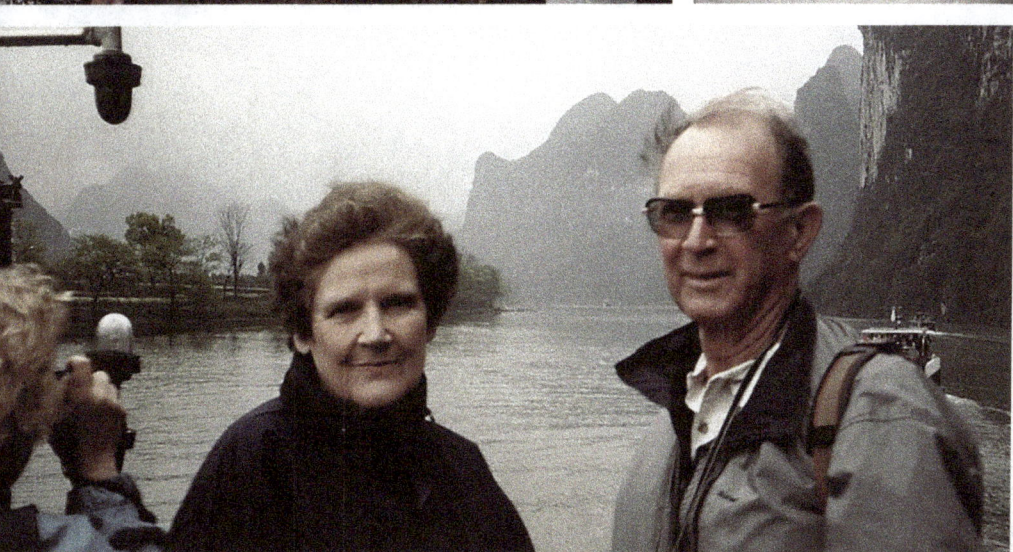
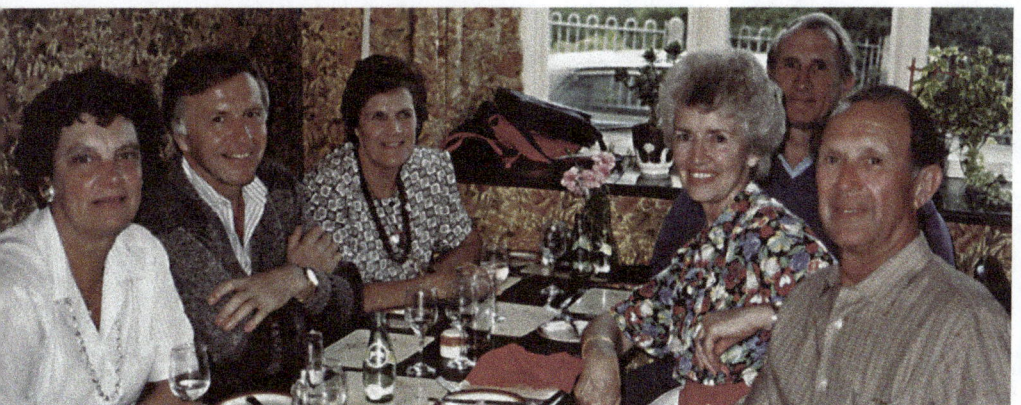

Clockwise: Fuff and June, Cahors, France 1995; June prepares bread from scratch in ancient flour mill, Cappodoccia, Turkey 1991; June & Errol river cruise, Li River, Guilin, China 1996; The Archdeacons hosting the Burdons & Cordners, Sidmouth, Devon, UK 1989.

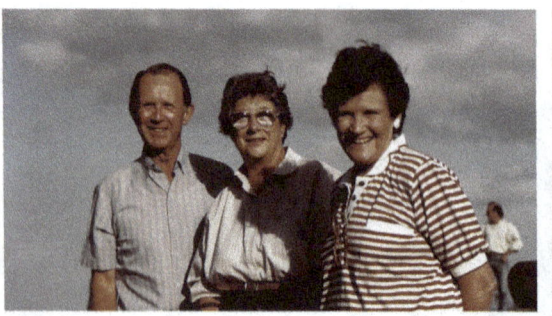
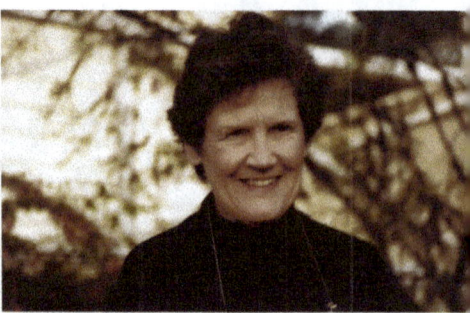
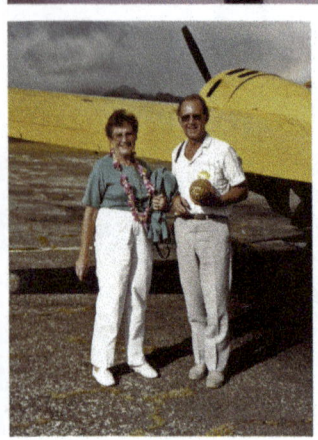
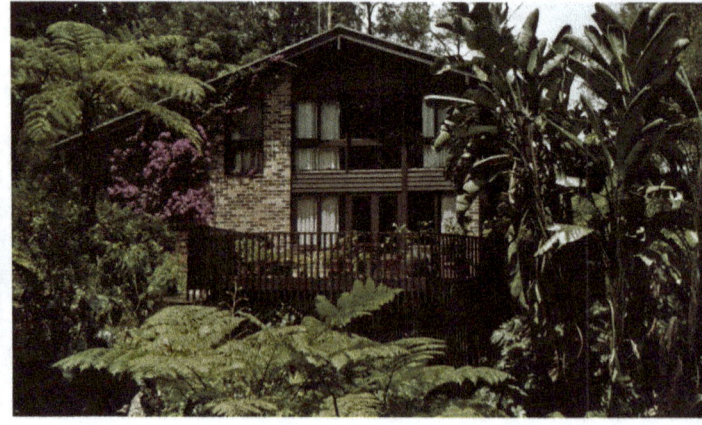

Clockwise: Errol, Dot Perry (widow of George) & June, Bateau Bay, NSW 1994; June 1992; June the Fearless, swims naked and runs Roaring Beach, Tas 1997; Forest home, Finlay Rd, Warrawee 1995; June & Errol took a joy flight around Hawaii 1989.

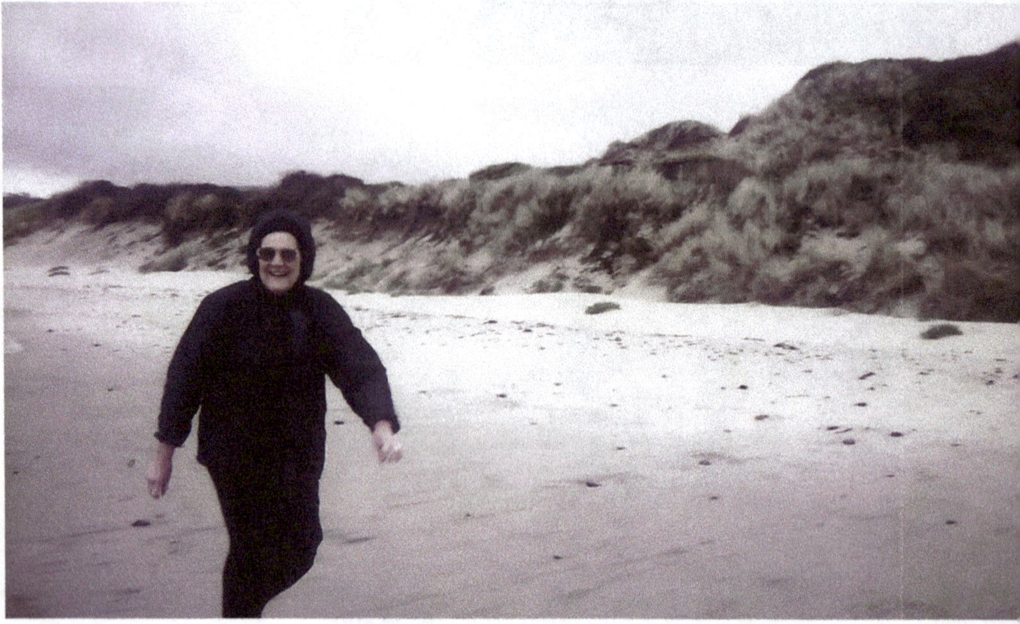

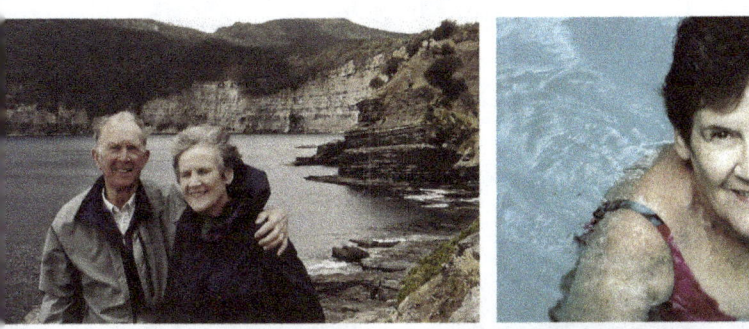
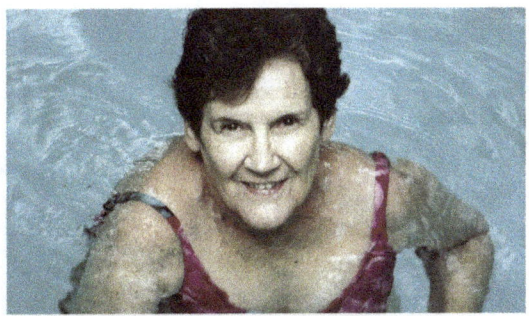
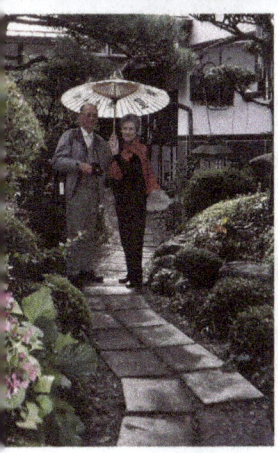
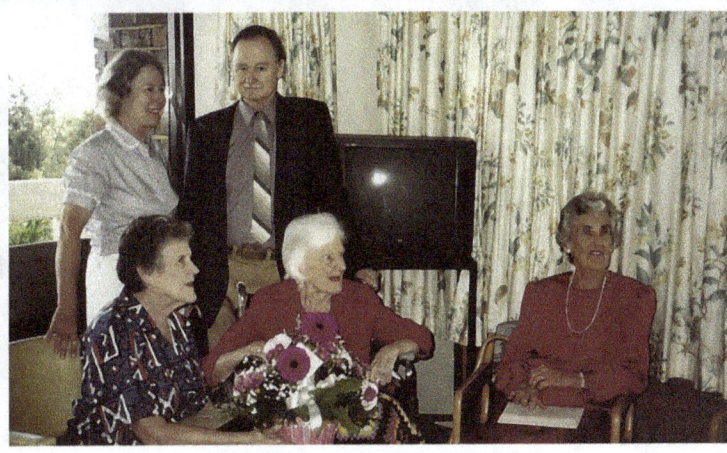

Clockwise: Errol & June, Maria Island, Tas 2000; June in pool, Finlay Rd, Warrawee c1998; June in front of Parliament, Budapest, Hungary 1999; June, John Miller and wife, Frances celebrate Aunt Jess' 100th birthday, Adelaide 1991; Errol & June in Aizuwakamatsu gardens, Japan 1998.

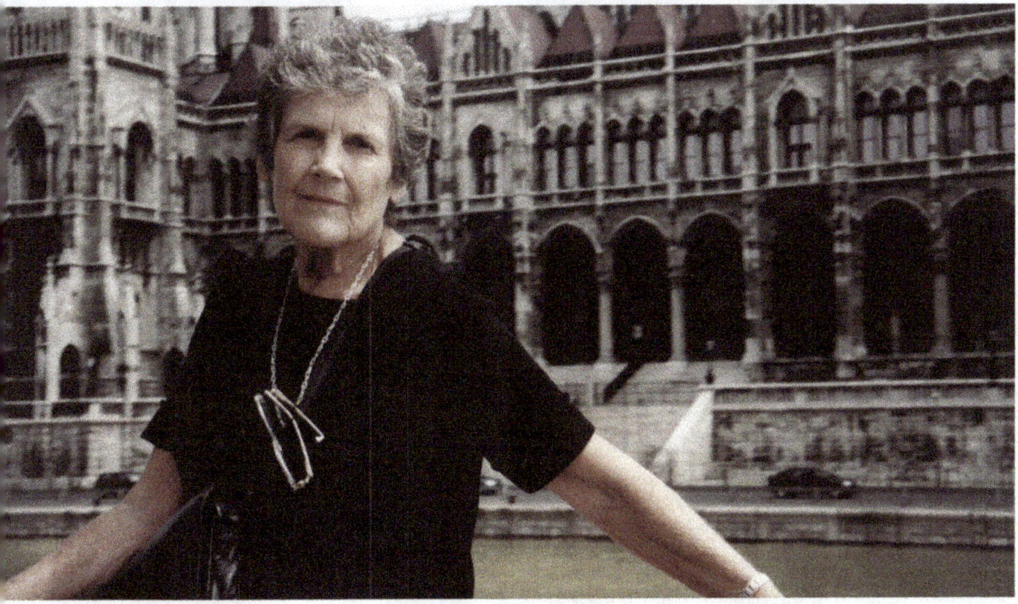

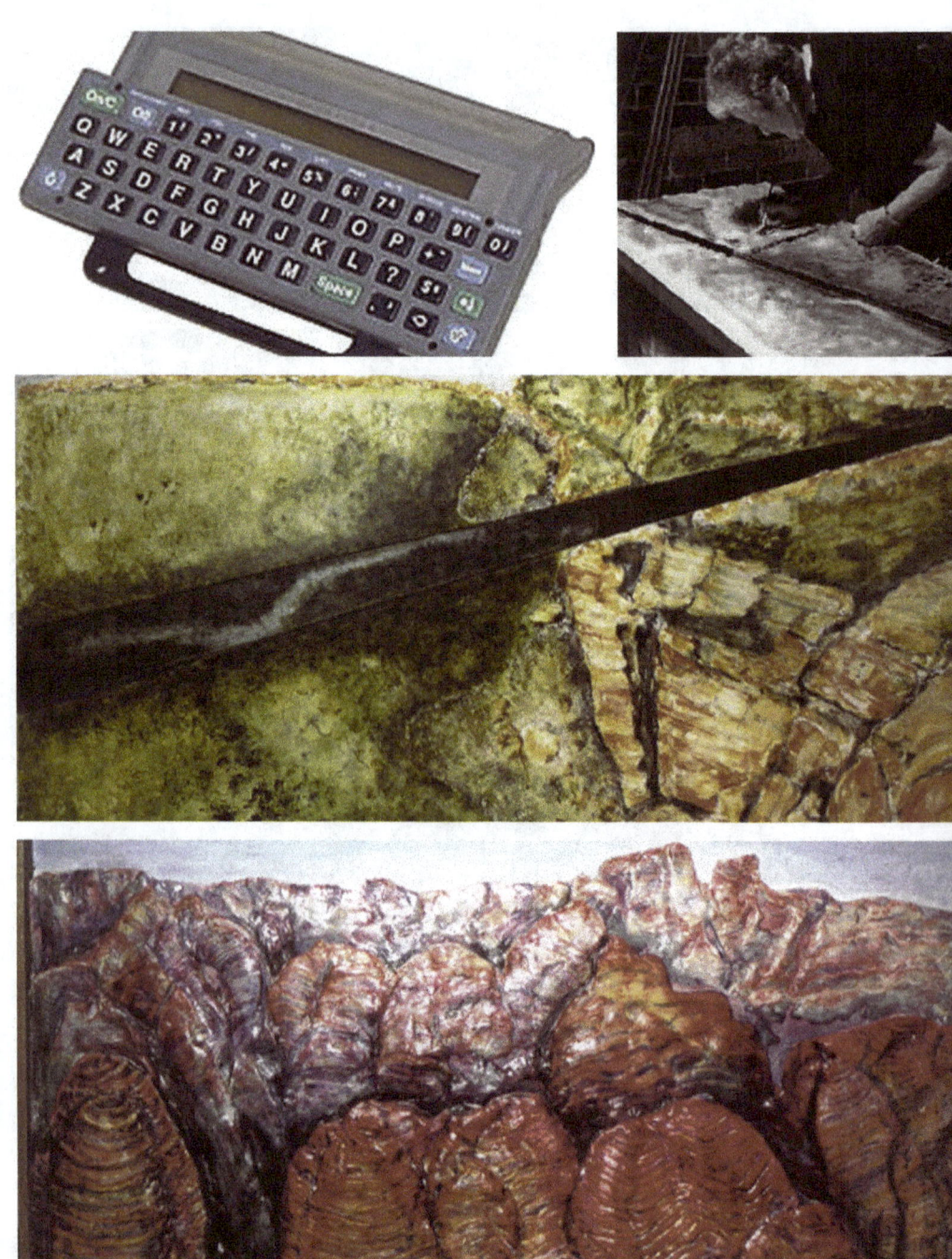

Clockwise: The Lightwriter displays text typed for the receiver and generates speech for phone calls as well, 2002; Artist at work on Wynne Submission, Finlay Rd garage, 2002; Kakadu Escarpment, Wynne Prize submission, Sydney 2001; Bungle Bungles, Wynne Prize submission, Sydney 2001.

Return to Australia

As our boys were growing older, we soon realised that we could not live in an apartment forever, and if we wanted to return to Australia we would have to make some definite plans. Errol mentioned our intentions to his boss at Canadian Car and Foundry, who immediately responded by saying he could possibly help us with a referral to the Chairman of Massey Ferguson - another Canadian company. As it happened, the Australian Comptroller was to be in Toronto the following week, and interviewed and hired Errol on the spot. The arrangement was that they would meet all expenses for our return, including furniture and belongings, and Errol was to start work in Melbourne as soon as possible.

The voyage home

Within six weeks, we were on the high seas aboard SS Orcades, travelling first class with a luxury cabin for us, and another for the boys. Thinking of it now, I cannot believe that the two little boys, aged two years and one year nine months, slept alone in their cabin. However, there was always a vigilant cabin steward, who doubtless checked regularly through the night, just as they did during our dinner and the evening entertainment. Many people travelled with children with the expectation, certainly in first class, that their little darlings would be cared for night and day. We supervised their meals and they spent the rest of the day in the fully equipped nursery with trained staff. One of the staff recounted an amusing anecdote, that once when a child started throwing sand at Trevor, Ross rushed to his defence and retaliated by throwing sand at the other boy. Ross maintained his defence on each subsequent day until the offender was kept away from the sandpit play area

It so happened that we were on the same ship as Anne and Wally Fotheringham with daughter Sarah, also returning to Australia. We sailed from Vancouver and had intended taking the train from east to west through the Rockies. Unfortunately, this did not eventuate because of an untimely train strike. Instead we flew, which was a nightmare. After a delayed departure from Montreal and a stopover in Toronto, it was an hour in the air before cabin staff would warm a bottle for a ravenous Ross, already hours overdue for his feed. Consequently, he cried for the entire flight and I was moved to the rear of the plane, nursing my screaming distressed child throughout the long night.

For two days, Lorne Hewson's brother entertained us. He showed us the sights of Vancouver, a beautiful city with a magnificent harbour and backdrop of snow-covered mountains. I was fascinated in Stanley Park by the beauty of the rich green velvety moss covering everything, something I had not seen growing on the east coast.

As frequently happens, for the first few days at sea many passengers suffer from seasickness, as did Errol, so I coped alone with the boys until reaching San Francisco. Together with the 'Foths' we took a day tour, visiting Hollywood Bowl, Gaumont Theatre and Fisherman's Wharf and other popular tourist spots. From a shop at the Wharf, I bought some inexpensive pearl shell earrings, which I wore on and off over the next forty years until sadly one was lost - putting paid to rest Errol's claim that I don't use such purchases! Actually, he is right most of the time. Next port of call was Hawaii and a day on Waikiki Beach, then on to Fiji and shopping for souvenirs at the markets where I purchased a huge woven reed basket, which I used as a sewing basket for twenty years. In 1960, Fiji was not a tourist destination and very different to what it is like today. As we approached the island and sailed alongside, we could see villages of native huts amidst the palms along the coastal beaches. Our last stop was Auckland before arriving in Australia and sailing into Sydney heads.

The entire voyage was a luxury holiday in every sense for us, with sports and evening entertainment, dancing, films, cards and fancy dress, and the children were well catered for at all times. Trevor and Ross won prizes in their fancy dress, for which they received bags of sweets. Like most children Ross disposed of his very quickly but we were intrigued by Trevor, who rationed himself to one sweet a day so they would last to be enjoyed for the rest of the voyage - amazing thinking for a child not yet three years.

One night Ross scared the wits out of the crew, and us, when we returned to the cabin to find his bed empty. After looking under the beds and every possible hiding place, we alerted the stewards, who continued looking outside the cabin without result. All was panic when despite the doors to the decks being too heavy for a child to open (even sturdy Ross!); it was presumed that he must have slipped through unseen with an adult. A full-scale search was mounted and the crew prepared to turn around the ship, as required when 'man overboard'. When someone decided to look again under his bed, there he was, sound asleep rolled into a little ball behind a small suitcase! Something had obviously upset him and only Ross could escape such detection.

Another incident, which did not end so happily, was when the ship did turn around to retrieve the body of a young man. He had been drunk and on being refused further drinks in the steerage bar, threatened to throw himself overboard, which he did. It takes an hour or so for a large liner to turn and to retrace its path, so he was long since dead. We watched with mixed emotions of fascination and horror, as the crew in a small lifeboat hauled his cold blue corpse aboard. Errol captured the body retrieval on film.

We celebrated Christmas 1960 on board, and I wore a beautiful peacock green, ruched taffeta skirt and bodice, thereafter christened my Christmas tree dress. Before departing Montreal, we had visited Midge and Norm in New York, where I had a shopping spree buying several cocktail dresses for the voyage.

A few days after Christmas, we sailed into Sydney Harbour but before doing so, we waited at the heads to allow the SS Orion on her maiden voyage, to enter first. We spent four days in Sydney over New Year and then sailed on to Melbourne where we disembarked. We then continued by train to Adelaide and a great reunion with family and friends. Errol had the romantic idea that it would be nice to come through the picturesque Adelaide hills and arrive by overnight train.

Not so pleasant though was our day continually swatting flies while waiting for the train. We were later to find out that there was a plague that year. I had forgotten about Aussie flies and felt like getting straight back on the ship, and back to Canada.

After a nine-year absence, I wanted to look my best on arrival in Adelaide. I wore a beautiful new cream suit and pillbox hat, a la Jackie Kennedy, which I had bought in Sydney at Anthony Horderns. The little boys were dressed in their cute tartan pants and, no doubt, Errol looked his usual smart self! It is amazing how one dressed up in those days. Fuff and Bob, who were then living in Port Adelaide, threw a welcome home party, after which we drove with Mum and Dad to Burra. A long hot drive as I recall. The boys and I stayed for a six weeks while Errol flew to Melbourne after a few days, to his new job and to look for a house where we would join him.

Melbourne and pregnant again

We had returned to Australia in January 1961, and were renting a big, furnished house in High Street, Mont Albert when in April I noticed I had missed a period. As Errol was unhappy at Massey Ferguson for various reasons, we were contemplating a change and a move to another State, preferably somewhere warmer as Melbourne was cold at that time, especially as there was no central heating.

It was not that we did not want another child but we had two small children and an uncertain future. Auntie Kath was staying with us and as a former nurse of the old school encouraged me to take hot baths, an old-fashioned method said to bring on the periods. Fortunately, the hot baths did nothing, for I was indeed pregnant and cannot imagine life without Jennifer. Jennifer was shocked on hearing that she was not a planned baby, which she interpreted as being not wanted. If all babies were planned, there would be fewer of them, as can be seen to be happening today in the western world. In our day, there was no effective contraceptive and there never really was a perfect time. It is like knowing the sex of an unborn child and, in my opinion, spoils the wonder and surprise element of creation.

I am very much against abortion. First and foremost, because I cannot imagine life without any of our three children, and had I undergone abortions I would have destroyed three potentially beautiful human beings. In my opinion saying that a foetus is not a living being is no argument, for if allowed to mature full term it takes on a human form. When faced with the untimely pregnancies, or so we selfishly thought, Dr Oxorn in Montreal had said he could refer patients to a doctor who practised abortions. Although I never asked him, he had also pointed out that he saw so many women who were desperate to have children and others who might conceive once, but never again. I also clearly remember an occasion in Montreal when my period was overdue and after going to the toilet, I was horrified to see a bloody rat-like creature in the toilet bowl. It was some time before I realised that it must be an aborted foetus. I was shocked to see that at a few weeks old it was not just a mass of blood and tissue, as I would have expected, but already showing some features and form. Whether animal or human, it was living, growing, and a part of me. I have never forgotten this experience. Lastly, we lost a daughter Petrina June (born 8th September 1963) at three months, who was also unplanned, and despite the fact that we do have three other children, I have never gotten over the sorrow of her death.

The house in Mont Albert was rented for twelve months and we had been looking to buy in Melbourne. However when the decision was made to change jobs and possibly move interstate, we had to move quickly on both counts if we were to be settled before the next baby arrived. The Massey Ferguson factory was north-west of Melbourne, in Sunshine, and was an hour by train or car. As it was too far for Errol to attend any interviews during the day, he resigned while looking for alternative employment. It was three months before he got another position at the right salary, and level of seniority, which appealed to him. In spite of our desire for a warmer climate, it was Tasmania, which was to be our home for the next eighteen years. Early October 1961, we made a rushed trip in our new automatic Ford Falcon to see my parents and other relatives. My mother had not been well for several years, and it was unlikely that she would ever make a trip to Tasmania.

Returning from Adelaide with car packed and our two little boys, we took the overnight ferry to Tasmania. Ann and Wally farewelled us, and after leaving Port Melbourne and land behind we went to the lounge. We ordered brandies with lemonade (there being no ginger ale) for Errol and me, and lemonade for the boys. Errol and I both remarked that the waiter was pretty light with the brandy, then realised that the waiter had mixed up our drinks, giving us lemonade and the boys the brandies! As it turned out, we were most grateful, for we had a peaceful and undisturbed night in spite of the rough seas of Bass Strait, Tasmania.

Tasmania

Early the next morning we disembarked at Devonport and drove along picturesque coastal road to Burnie. We were booked in at the best hotel in the town, The Menai, which was owned and run by 'Wif' Campbell and his wife. The hotel itself was quite comfortable but I am sure that the TV series 'Faulty Towers' was based on this hotel and its owners. The guests were a nuisance, who interfered with the Campbell's lives. The two and a half months we spent as their 'guests' were at times a nightmare and at other times hilariously funny. I must add their behaviour was not at all typically Tasmanian and despite all disparaging remarks made by other Australians about the Taswegians, I found that on the whole they were more hospitable, well educated, and interesting than anywhere else I have been. Our recollections of ridiculous events would fill a book.

Soon after our arrival we were welcomed by Margaret Minns, who with husband Derek and their children Nicky and Sarah, were also resident at the hotel since their recent arrival from England. Derek was the newly appointed Assistant General Manager of Tioxide Australia, where Errol was to be employed as Chief Accountant, and later as Commercial Manager of the company. The Minns had the hotel's only suite and each afternoon and sometimes morning when we were at home, Margaret invited me to her lounge where we would sip tea and gossip while the boys would play with Sarah, aged four. One thing which stands out in my memory, is Margaret marvelling at Ross' skill and compassion at two and a half, in catching blowflies trapped inside the glass window and allowing them to fly free through an open window. To this day macho Ross goes to great lengths to free any insect caught inside the house.

Margaret and I got on well together, as indeed did Errol and Derek. Their son Nicky, then aged six, and Sarah loved to look after our two little boys. One day young Nicky in all earnestness asked Derek, as he was the Assistant General Manager why didn't he make Uncle Errol the

General Manager of the company! The following months and especially at weekends, our two families went for drives to various beauty spots nearby. Once settled in our own homes most Sundays were spent picnicking at the beach, and Errol and Derek played golf on Saturdays. This continued for the three years that the Minns lived in Burnie, before their return to Britain.

Early on, much of our time was spent house hunting in Burnie and nearby Ulverstone, a pretty little town where many of the senior staff lived. The factory and staff offices were situated at Chasm Creek two miles east of Burnie, with Ulverstone further to the east. There were a few small company houses at Chasm Creek close to the factory, and high on the hill behind stood the newly built General Manager's company home with extensive gardens. It had been recently occupied by Herbert Nicholls (Nick) and Frances and their family, son Patrick, and daughters Helen, Jane, Josephine (Jo), and nine months later Margaret (Meg). The home was large enough for a big family and suitable for entertaining directors visiting from the British parent company. Frances was an excellent and untiring hostess, and with the assistance of one or two women gave wonderful lunches and dinner parties for visitors, newcomers and the wives of leading locals. In fact, I believe it was she who was responsible in many ways for a happy and loyal senior staff. She was a capable organiser and an active chairwoman of many local charities. By contrast, Nick though popular with his employees was a shy and retiring man. Shortly after our arrival, we were invited to a dinner party to meet the Directors and their wives, and a luncheon was held for me to meet some of Frances' closest woman friends. Strangely enough, among them were our immediate neighbours and my future friends.

Every year on the first Tuesday in November, Melbourne Cup day, she invited about forty women for lunch, and to watch the horse race on TV. Australians love to place bets on this special day and parties like these take place all over Australia. All the women were decked out in brand new clothes and hats, as was the custom and one rarely wore the same outfit twice with the same group of women! There were so many social functions, which required dressing up, that life was never dull - though it was rather expensive. I loved clothes, and fortunately, Errol was never mean and liked me to look attractive. Hats were no problem as there was an excellent hat shop in Burnie, and as well as stocking beautiful hats, the lady made hats to match any outfit. Consequently I had numerous hats, and day and evening frocks. As well as buying clothes off the rack, I found an excellent and very clever dressmaker who designed whatever I wanted. When Errol bought me a peacock green silk sari bordered with gold from Thailand, she wisely talked me out of making an evening frock from it, which would have wasted yards of the long sari and lost most of the gold border. Instead she made a long slip and a blouse of matching material, which her daughter delicately trimmed with gold thread around the neckline and short sleeves. And so I wore the sari as it is meant to be worn, and as is the case with all saris, they can be worn by any woman no matter what her age or size. I still have this beautiful and quite valuable sari, which our daughter may wish to wear someday.

Many people were in awe of Frances, even her friends of long-standing confessed this, and so to be on her guest list was special. As I was a few years younger and she was the wife of Errol's boss, I addressed her as Mrs Nicholls, as one did in those days. Once we became more familiar, she asked me to call her Frances and from then on, we considered ourselves friends. She is a very loyal friend, always writing and phoning, and never fails to contact us when she is in Sydney. She is truly a remarkable and independent woman, and still travels a lot. As she recently said, life could be very lonely if she didn't keep in touch with all her old friends and be prepared to keep a full life. Nick died tragically well over thirty years ago, when driving down their steep drive his jeep went over the side. Neither he nor the jeep was found for several days. He had the habit of bushwalking alone for days, and as Frances was in Hobart at the time, she was not worried by his absence when she returned.

25 Seaview Avenue

The number of houses for sale was limited in the district and after some weeks, we eventually decided on the first one we had looked at. Twenty-five Seaview Avenue sat high on the hill on the western side of the town, with a magnificent view of the hills to the west, and the sea on two sides. We had the most glorious sunsets. The house was two storied with terraced lawns all around, bordering garden beds, a fishpond and many steps from the street to the front of the house, which continued around the side to the back. Ross will know how many steps, as he used to run down and up at the speed of sound to collect the morning paper. The natural stonewalls between the terraced lawns and steps had all been done by the previous owner Lloyd Harris, and were most attractive. In fact, the entire house and garden layout were all built by him. At the back, we had access from Grandview Avenue, where there was parking for our cars and a garden leading down to an enclosed paved area at the rear of the house.

It was an interesting layout and an open design with large windows, all with views. The back entrance and passage led straight into a laundry area with a toilet to the left, and bathroom and separate shower on the right. The passage continued straight ahead into the kitchen and as well to the left, to the main bedroom and another, which was to be our new baby's room. There was a door from the kitchen into the dining/lounge room, which in turn led into the sunroom at the front. There were extensive views of the garden and we overlooked the houses on the lower side of Seaview Avenue, the trees of Burnie Park and then beyond to the hills and Bass Strait to Table Cape. (Called Table Cake by Jennifer when she was little). This was to be my favourite room and became our living room where we spent most of our time day and night, looking at the view, watching TV or whatever. There was a large fireplace where we had roaring log fires, before and even after we had ducted heating installed. On the same wall in the lounge room there was another large fireplace, which effectively warmed most of the house. The front door on the bottom floor led into the entrance hall and at that time only one room, which became the boys' bedroom. We later added a full bathroom, and the next owners wisely added another bedroom as we had always planned. From the entrance, a wide stairway led up to the main living area and thence to the kitchen and upstairs bedrooms. With the exception of kitchen, bathroom and utility areas, all floors were natural Tasmanian myrtle, highly polished and very beautiful. We bought two large off-white Indian rugs for the dining/lounge room and off-white drapes for the large windows at either end and entrance hall. The boys and visiting children loved to slide around and I spent much time polishing. A few years later, for warmth and less work, we had the stairs and timber floors covered with wall-to-wall brown carpet. Unusual at that time, it looked most attractive with off-white drapes and walls. I hated covering the timber, and must add that at first the carpet man blatantly refused to do the dining/lounge room, as said he had never seen such beautiful timber floors all complemented by the off-white rugs, drapes and walls, and brown velvet lounge suite! In fact, he said it was a sacrilege to cover any of the timber, which indeed it was. We agreed with his suggestion that he do all floors, except that room, and that if we desired he would return and do it later. Although it looked nice, it proved impractical and we had the carpet installed throughout. More than twenty years later, the carpet was like new and I never got tired of the colour scheme. Much later, when we were moving out and the house was bereft of furniture, it all looked so nice and inviting that I wished I were moving in instead of out! On one return trip to Tasmania when visiting the present owners, Brian and Marlene Adams, I declared that I had never seen a more lovely home, together with the garden and view.

There were many other features that appealed to us. In most rooms there was built-in timber furniture, all beautifully crafted by Lloyd, so we had very little to buy. Nothing at all was required for our bedroom where there was a double bed with lamps on the headboard shelf and cupboards either side, wall-to-wall 'his and hers' wardrobes, and shelves and drawers in the middle. On an adjacent wall was a fitted dressing table with mirror and long corner chest of drawers. I believe all timber was silky oak, which had a light, soft sheen. In sunroom and lounge, there were cupboards and bookshelves on either side of the fireplaces and in the lounge a built-in seat. The sunroom had a movable lounge with cushions, which could be used as a bed, a small padded seat used for toy storage, and beside it a corner table with a reading lamp installed. In the dining area was a buffet, and the kitchen had a built-in table with cushioned seats either side, and storage underneath. In the passage, there was a huge linen cupboard with heated racks for drying. Also by the upstairs bedrooms was a cupboard in the wall for soiled clothes, the other side of which opened into the laundry. The children all had great fun hiding in this and Jennifer always expressed a desire to sleep in it. Finally we allowed her to fulfil this wish, but I think it maybe have been a short night. Another great hiding place was behind things in a cupboard under the stairs. Needless to say, we have missed all this storage space since we moved away, and our 'children' fortunately have long since got over their desire to hide when they visit us!

Another attraction was the huge area under the house, where everything was stored from golf clubs and wine to bicycles. Travelling trunks held my out-dated glamorous dresses, and Jennifer and Margaret Nicholls spent hours dressing up. We were to learn many years later that they sampled the sherry stored there as well.

Shortly after we bought the house, the Harris' had a large party to celebrate Lloyd's fortieth birthday and they kindly invited us to join them so we could meet our new neighbours and some of their friends. As mentioned before, I had met several of the women and we both had met a few of the men.

While living at the Menai we were invited to a few of our future friends' homes. On first arriving in the town, I promised to ring someone on the Sunday to make plans. As there was no-one in attendance at hotel reception, after 7 p.m. on weekdays and all weekend, the phone connection to the guests' rooms was cut off and one was expected to use the public call box in the foyer. However when I went to the phone in the foyer, it too did not work, so I rang the bell at reception. Mrs Campbell appeared and demanded to know what I wanted, and when told the reason said that it too was disconnected at the weekends. What was I to do, as I had to make a call? She declared that there was a phone box a few streets away, and refused my request to use her phone as it was not her problem. Then to my utter amazement and almost in tears, she added, 'Do you think I am just here every day at your beck and call? This is my home and I have a life too!' This was in spite of the fact that Tioxide was paying them very well for the Minns and our family. As well, throughout the year, the company had numerous visitors from interstate and overseas who stayed there. In the main, it was salesmen who stayed in the hotel, so it was usually quiet over weekends. Despite their reported wealth, the Campbells were very mean, and though they owned a timber mill, they refused our pleas to light the log fire in the guest lounge before 5 p.m. - no matter how cold or bleak the weather. We had an ally in Louis, the headwaiter cum handy man, who would light it when 'Mrs C' was not around. The most incredible and inhospitable time was when all the top tennis players in the world, including Hoad and Rosewall, were touring Australia giving demonstration matches and stayed at the Menai. One night at dinner, they were sitting at the next table and we overheard one of the Americans ask for some bread. We cringed with embarrassment and disbelief when he was told that only fairy bread (Melba toast) was served with dinner. The Minns eventually moved to the new Emu Motel and we would have done so too except that they had no adjoining rooms. Besides, we were reasonably comfortable with three good meals and two bedrooms - both with en-suites opposite each other. Once they got to sleep, the boys were sleeping through the night; they knew where to find us.

The boys were very well behaved in the dining room but as children were not allowed for dinner, they were fed in their bedroom. This was always a rush as their meal often arrived late, and it was difficult to settle them down before seven thirty, which was the deadline for dining - no excuses. Sometimes the boys had not settled, but when we checked later were always content or asleep. Unbeknown to us we later found out from other guests, who were drinking in the public lounge, that the boys frequently came out and entertained them before retiring. I think the boys may have been encouraged, as they looked very cute in their Canadian bunny rabbit pyjamas, with feet all in one, a fashion not yet in Australia. One night there was a great kerfuffle when a waiter came rushing into the dining room. The boys had appeared because one of them had gone into the bathroom and turned on a tap but could not turn it off. By the time help arrived, the entire bedroom was swamped. Surprisingly the Campbells were not at all perturbed and a team set about drying it out. When it was declared thoroughly dry (though the carpet still smelled), the boys were allowed back in without any suggestion of a change of room. What is more, there was no talk of the ruined carpet or even a charge on the bill! We ceased to be surprised.

Jennifer joins us

On the 19th December 1961, we moved into our very first home. Errol had already engaged the services of a young girl, Louise Bryant, who was the eldest of a large family of boys. She proved to be most capable and hard working. All through my pregnancy, I had kept very fit and well, and the baby was now overdue. The Minns were already settled in their home on Cunningham Street, which was close to the hospital, and so the following day the boys and I spent the day with Margaret. Late in the afternoon I felt the first contractions, and when Derek came home, he took me to the hospital. As the hospital was undergoing renovations all was in chaos. The admittance desk was unattended and no one appeared when he rang the bell, nor was there anyone in sight. It was really rather funny as he roamed the corridors calling, 'Is there anyone around? A lady here is about to give birth', which brought a rushed response from all directions and a reprimand for Derek when it was ascertained that it was not an emergency. The birth was not imminent and I was sent off to the labour ward. There was more confusion when it was established that Derek was not Mr Burdon, nor was he the father of the unborn child. In the meantime,

Errol had arrived at the Minns, collected the boys and taken them home to be in the care of Louise. Derek stayed with me until the arrival of Errol. Just before midnight 20th December 1961, and attended by Dr Tom Ingram the local obstetrician, I gave birth to our darling seven-pound-ten-ounce daughter - soon to be named Jennifer Margaret. She was always and still is called Jennifer by the family and school friends. When she was little and obviously aware of the Queen, she referred to herself as Jennifer Margaret Elizabeth Mary, and on occasions still does when phoning or signing letters or emails. Aged eighteen when she started university, she was immediately called Jenni - the name by which she is generally known now.

Jennifer and I spent our first Christmas together in Burnie General Hospital, and Errol and the boys with the Minns family. Many following Christmases were celebrated in the company of the Minns at either their home or ours. Although I had told Dr Ingram that my paediatrician in Montreal suggested I not attempt to breast-feed any future babies, this advice was ignored. After putting up with a very hungry baby, she too was finally put on the time-consuming routine of breast milk supplemented with cow's milk in a bottle, which continued for three months after I went home. Following their paediatrician's advice both the boys at eight weeks were given canned baby food, initially a teaspoon of banana, slowly increasing in quantity and progressing to vegetable and some weeks later to a little meat. However, the nurse from the Burnie Baby Health Clinic, who visited, was horrified at the mere suggestion and insisted I continue with the milk diet for some months. I did so for a while to please her until I reasoned that the boys had thrived and were healthy, and that I would make my own judgement.

Burnie was a busy port and thriving town when we arrived. The two major employers were Australian Pulp and Paper Mill (APPM) and Australian Tioxide, the former having the larger workforce. Thirty years on APPM have closed much of their plant, and in the mid-nineties, Tioxide closed down altogether. Consequently, the young people are leaving for want of work and the town has been in slow decline. Lactos Cheese factory, started by a Dutch migrant Milan Vynalek and his wife, was a two-man work force in the late fifties and after growing and expanding was bought out twenty years later by the French company Bongrain. It now exports its excellent cheeses all over the world. There are few other such companies in the area and it is not the centre it once was. When we last returned, however, we were most impressed by the many improvements in the business centre, along the seafront and to the town in general. It looked like a very progressive town, not one in decline. For the time we lived there, it was an excellent and happy environment to raise a family, and still is I believe.

We were delighted with our home, all spick and span, floors all highly polished by the capable Miss Bryant, who could not continue with us, as she was needed at home. Through Peggy Gill, who lived with husband David across the road, I obtained the services of the wonderful Maude Masters. Maudie as she preferred to be called, even by the children, was an absolute treasure and became more than a friend to us all. She loved children and treated ours as her own, especially Jennifer, who was her baby. She spent three mornings housekeeping and cooking for elderly neighbours where she sometimes slept. She cleaned for the Gills and two days came to me. She made herself available at other times and was willing to sleep overnight. Maudie was never idle as she would always iron or cook meals and biscuits on these overnight stays, when she was happy to sleep on the sofa bed in the sunroom. She was a spinster and being a devout Baptist, her life was dedicated to her work and helping people. She had a knitting machine on which she made woollens for overseas missions, and happily made many jumpers for the boys, for which we paid. It was hard to tell her age but she was tiny, and had the appearance of an outdoor country person used to hard work. She must have been in her late fifties when she first came to us, as she died about twenty years ago when approaching ninety.

Our life was full with our small family. Very soon, I felt that I must repay the hospitality extended to me by women in the district. I did so by having two luncheons, serving the same menu for twelve in two consecutive weeks. I loved cooking and chose some unusual dishes for that time in Australia. I baked an orange glazed ham, surrounded by garnished baked pears and peaches, curries, and various vegetable and jellied savoury salads. For dessert, I prepared lemon meringue pie, the delicious pumpkin chiffon pie (new to Australian palates), my colourful cassata icecream, and finished with cheeses and coffee. I still remember the menu, as I had to be well organised and wrote it out as part of my preparation. Maudie helped in the kitchen and afterwards commented that she could not believe how much noise twelve women could make with their chatter!

Many such luncheon and dinner parties followed over the years and proved to be a very successful way of introducing new people to the area. As well, there were many neighbourly coffee mornings and it was rare for a week to pass without assisting or attending a charity event - usually at a private home. We baked, supplied produce, and knitted and sewed articles for the trading table. This was a costly business after paying entrance, buying raffle tickets and making purchases from the trading table - often for things that we did not need! I once suggested, half seriously, that we would make more money if we all donated five pounds a week and save us a lot of work. Frances, who had a vast vegetable and flower garden tended by the company gardener, ridiculed this idea, but the rest did not have this advantage. To prove my point I decided to calculate what I spent and discovered that it could be well over twenty pounds, especially by the time I included child minding.

I joined Red Cross, the Young Victoria League, and the Baby Heath Centre of which Margaret soon became President. When she returned to England, I took over as President, during which time we held a big fund-raising luncheon and fashion parade at Breckenborough House - a lovely reception home. This was a great success but as I had made a speech (my first ever) in front of more than a hundred people, I was relieved when it was over. I rehearsed it well and though my knees were shaking, it was delivered with no apparent nervousness - or so I was told.

Despite living right on the coast with beaches everywhere, it was the custom for many of our friends to sojourn to Boat Harbour Beach for the summer and other holidays. Many had their own holiday cottages (shacks) and others rented. For our first few summers, together with the Minns, we rented at Eleanor Cottages. They were run by George and Rex, two charming and rather eccentric homosexuals, who were excellent hosts. They held dinner parties on their terrace for us and each course was served with great flourish. We can never forget the tantrum Rex, always the prima donna, threw when serving the lobster cocktail and, horror of horrors, discovered that one cocktail was short of a claw garnish! No words could console him and the dinner was almost cancelled until Margaret finally convinced him to give her the clawless one ... and she would make believe she had two claws. Margaret became quite a favourite with the boys, especially Rex, who had a background in amateur theatre, as did she. In fact, the boys on later visits to the UK made good use of the Minns' hospitality, rather overstaying their welcome on one occasion. These enjoyable dinners came to an abrupt end, when health inspectors found their kitchen was not tiled to health standards and their licence was cancelled.

We whiled away our days on the beach with our friends carrying on from where we left off at home - a little Burnie away from home. Our days were fully occupied swimming, sunning ourselves while the children played, and walking to the rock pool or out along the headland. Surprisingly, none of the children was deterred by the cold water. Families gathered for beach picnics and pre-dinner drinks at night, while some of the men fished and distributed their catches to other families. I remember little curly haired Chris Clarke, now a well-known ABC foreign correspondent, coming around selling fish for pocket money. Many years later, I taught Chris art at Burnie High School and recall that his father was a journalist for the local paper, The Advocate. One day when our boys were perhaps six and five, they disappeared with Andrew Gill, then seven years old. They had told someone that they were going to see Andrew's Nanna and set off along the coast towards Wynyard some ten miles away. Panic set in and the men went searching for the wayward boys. They were found unharmed but well on their way towards some perilous cliffs.

During these years Trevor, who was always very exact, came out with some famous lines. Once when at Boat Harbour beach, Nick asked him what I was doing. Trevor replied, 'I don't know Mr Nicholls, I'm down here on the beach and she's up there at the shack.' Also, two instances when Maudie, who thought Trevor was perfect, remarked that he was getting a little bit rude. He had been playing with his little Dinky toy car on the laminex table when she told him not to run the car and scratch the table. His reply was, 'But I am not scratching the table, Maudie.' The other occasion was when she asked him to run and fetch something, which he did, and was then told not to run in the house! How confusing is adult speech to a child? How often do we say such things and after they take us literally, we reprimand them? When Trevor started school, our next-door neighbour John Gandy brought him home when he picked up his daughter Pam. On their way home, John and Pam usually called in to see John's elderly mother. One evening Trevor asked, 'How long is a minute Daddy? Mr Gandy always says, "We will only be a minute Trevor" but I am always waiting so long?'

Petrina June ... briefly

In January 1963 when at Boat Harbour, I found I was again pregnant. This was bad timing as I already had my hands full with three little ones aged three and under, while Errol was busy at work and doing a lot of travelling. Nature had her way however and on 8th September 1963, Petrina June joined the Burdon clan, making the perfect family of two boys and two girls - all under five years. For some reason when in hospital I felt this baby was very special and precious, which is not to say that the others were not but it was different when I cuddled Petrina. The birth was quite normal and Dr Ingram pronounced her quite healthy. Once again in hospital, despite my protestations, the sister in charge insisted I breastfeed, which proved as unsuccessful as before. Once home I endured hours on end, both night and day, trying to satisfy a hungry crying babe and at the same time had three other little ones to care for. The visiting Baby Health Sister declared Petrina perfectly healthy but to me it was obvious all was not well. On our next check up with Tom Ingram, I expressed my concerns but he could not discern anything wrong. He added that he did not know much about newborn babies and would refer me to a paediatrician in Launceston. Friday of the following week Errol, Petrina, and I set off for our appointment. I sat in the back with Petrina and, on the way, she suddenly turned blue, which increased my anxiety greatly. We arrived at the doctor's surgery in time for the twelve o'clock appointment, and after examining her, he quickly diagnosed her as having a congenital 'hole in the heart'. He reassured us that unlike other heart conditions, she was in no danger of suddenly dropping dead. She would require several small feeds throughout the day in order to receive sufficient nutrition, and in two to three years could have surgery to correct the condition. I knew all about this as my sister Helen's youngest, Diana also had a hole in the heart and had undergone several successful operations. Although he was not concerned about her, he said he would like to put her in hospital as there was a heart specialist coming from Melbourne the following Monday. We agreed and arrived at the hospital at one o'clock. It was four o'clock before Petrina was admitted and still had not been fed since leaving home early that morning. We had her bottle, which had only had to be warmed, and a tin of powdered soymilk to use as substitute for cow's milk. We finally left at six o'clock believing our baby was in safe hands and with the knowledge that we could return if necessary in a couple of hours. We collected the children from the Minns, who persuaded us to have dinner, as we had not eaten all day. On arriving home, there was a message at the exchange saying our baby was seriously ill with pneumonia. Some weeks later a Sister, who had come on duty at seven o'clock that same evening, said what callous parents we must be to leave the hospital when our baby was so ill. We also learned that she had been christened that same night.

Thereafter tragic though it was, the next two weeks was a travesty of errors. In the following days, we were told to ring at regular times and to speak with Petrina's doctor. Often he was not available and we spoke to the sisters-in-charge, who told us varying things from day to day. Such as: she was much improved; worse; had put on weight (to an impossible figure way above her admission weight); drinking well; that her pneumonia was under control; had turned for the worse or improved ... and so it went on. As requested we rang on Monday to see what the heart specialist had said, only to be told that the neither the specialist nor paediatrician had seen her. They seemed to have forgotten all about her, and to not know what we were talking about. They were both going to Hobart for a week, to a conference, and could not be contacted. At this time Errol's mother, who had been living in Kalgoorlie, WA, was seriously ill with brain cancer and in a Perth Hospital. After a week, finally we were told that Petrina had turned the corner and was recovering, and that we should not worry. Errol flew to Perth late Friday, checked on Petrina's condition early Saturday when the report was good, not so good early Sunday but again a glowing report of impossible gain in weight late Sunday. It was a nightmare.

At seven o'clock, when still in bed, I received a phone call from the hospital, a nurse simply advising me that our baby had died. I was alone at home with three small children, and not knowing what to do I phoned the Minns, who helped contact Errol. Soon after I received another call, asking what I wanted done with the body as it could not stay in their morgue. Derek sought advice from our local doctor Ed Barron, who made the necessary arrangements to transfer her to a funeral parlour. It was all quite inhumane; the number of phone calls I received within a few hours of her death, none of which I could answer without Errol. To add to this the account for services rendered arrived from the paediatrician the following week! As soon as he could get a flight, a distraught Errol arrived home. We were then faced with the dilemma of what to do with our tiny baby, and whether to arrange a burial or cremation. As we did not expect to stay forever in Burnie, or even in Tasmania, I hated the idea of leaving our little daughter alone in some faraway place never to be visited by family. Dear Maudie suggested Penguin cemetery on the hill, overlooking the sea and she promised to visit every week. On the other hand, the thought of cremating a three month old was equally abhorrent. Despite these misgivings and because we both believed in cremation, we decided on that option. The Friday following Petrina's death, Errol and I set off on our sad journey for Launceston to be reunited with Petrina for the last time. On the way I told Errol of my thoughts about adopting a baby, which I felt would give some meaning to Petrina's short life on earth and as well, give a home to another child. Errol did not want to talk about it, saying it was not the time to discuss it, and mine was just a natural emotional reaction after losing a baby. (Actually, this was not the case, as I had always wanted to adopt a child.) Besides he said, we could not afford it, forgetting that had she lived we would have managed to afford her, not to mention the fact that we were comfortably well off! The topic was not raised or discussed again. Ironically, thirty years later we met a lovely dark-haired girl (as was Petrina), who was born the same day as Petrina and had been adopted by a couple in north-eastern Tasmania.

On arrival at the funeral parlour, we were led into a small chapel where Petrina lay in her tiny coffin. When I leaned over to kiss her, I was surprised by how cold and hard she felt - just like marble. In an instant my fears about cremating this tiny being disappeared, I knew that nothing could hurt her now. It was a heart-wrenching moment and the first time that I had seen Errol cry when we said a prayer and bid our farewells. The funeral director suggested that her ashes be spread in the nearby park, to which we agreed, and as we were too upset to think about any details, no arrangements for any remembrance have ever been made. She is truly forgotten as a part of our lives and it is as though she never existed. She died on the 13th of November 1963, aged nine weeks. What is sadder is that we don't even have any photos. The others were all much photographed but for some reason Petrina missed out. I do recall a photo being taken on a picnic with my cousin Dee, who had come from Melbourne to assist with the other children, but it has never been found. Driving home in silence after the service, we were both very emotional. We collected the children and from the next day on life continued on the surface as it had before Petrina. As for me, I was kept busy with home, family and my other interests; I did not grieve openly, nor have I since. I have found this very difficult, as I have needed to talk about it.

Settled for eighteen years

Trevor started kindergarten at Burnie Primary School when aged five. There was a ridiculous policy that children were not allowed to learn the alphabet or to read until six years of age, and although he was almost six, this rule applied to him. He was extremely bright and anxious to learn, and could already read and count. In fact, the latter he had virtually taught himself. One morning Errol got up to find Trevor sitting at the kitchen table with an encyclopaedia. Trevor proudly announced, 'Daddy I can now, count and write to one thousand.' He had been right through the book patiently copying the numbers from each page - he certainly used his initiative. We have another delightful story from the time we were living in Melbourne and when Errol bought him a colouring-in book. Trevor was only three and after spending hours colouring a dozen or so pictures, he suddenly put down his crayons and said, 'I'm so tired, I can't finish today.' The dear little fellow thought that he had to finish the book.

Ross was equally bright and took every opportunity to learn. I remember thinking that neither need go to school as they could educate themselves, especially when Ross in second year high school was home convalescing after hurting his leg playing his first game of rugby,. He spent all and every day reading Encyclopaedia Britannica. At the same time his then Maths teacher sent home ten problems, which she said would challenge her star pupil, as some of the HSC (Higher School Certificate) teachers said it should keep Ross occupied for some days. Well, after a few hours of my giving it to Ross, both he and Trevor, and not to mention Errol had solved each problem! At a very early age, both boys learned a lot about figures and language from Errol, as did

Jennifer. When she is unsure of the correct grammar, which is not really taught in schools now, she still refers to Errol. He is fanatical about correct usage and the way the English language is abused today. Errol cannot read a business letter without correcting the grammar or spelling, and when watching TV cannot resist commenting on the constant misuse of language, particularly by the so-called educated leaders of the community.

All our children are avid readers and I was amazed at the books Trevor brought home from the library on every conceivable subject: judo, modelling aeroplanes, mathematical problems, chess, the solar system, wizardry and so the list went on satisfying his lust for learning. Ross was very much into science fiction when young and has since progressed to deeper topics, and what I would call philosophical texts, as well as a love of poetry, and classical and modern music. Jennifer too has a taste for all manner of subjects, classics and modern. When they were in primary school, a friend once remarked that children were not encouraged to read books anymore as her children did no reading, which surprised me because our three literally devoured books. In their term report cards, their level of reading was always at least five years above the average, whereas I believed they were only average.

Trevor and Ross both excelled in primary school, topping their respective classes with little competition and continuing in this vein in high school. Their IQ tests disclosed scores of over 140, and also placed Jennifer in the superior range. Judging by the children I taught and their IQ rankings, I am led to believe that if 100 is average, then the average person is pretty daft and not really capable of handling the complexities of reading and writing English or problem solving. Although such persons may function very well at many jobs as they did in years gone by, they are not lateral thinkers as required in most business situations nowadays. When I was teaching I came across no more than ten students out of two thousand (0.5 per cent), who had an IQ of 100 or less - so where are the other 49.5 per cent? I want to stress that this is only my personal observation but it seemed that average IQ was more like 120.

Both boys were selected by the headmaster, Alan Thorne, to represent Burnie Primary School on various occasions including the Anzac Day service in West Park. Ross read a passage from the Bible at a Christmas radio broadcast, and we were surprised to hear it, as he had not told us beforehand. On entering high school, Trevor received the prize for the most outstanding student from Burnie Primary, a prize that was discontinued the following year. Their years at Burnie High were happy and successful, receiving dux of class and winning Science and Maths prizes each year. Both were recommended for Rotary and American Field Scholarships, but were not keen to leave their friends and delay their entry to university. Trevor later expressed his regret at this, as he realised that such scholarships can open many doors in the future. He was selected as the first Tasmanian schoolboy to qualify for a year's attendance at an overseas International English School. We literally had to push him on the plane for his final interview in Melbourne, with a panel of three headed by Sir Garfield Barwick, the much-respected High Court Judge. As the destination was to be Singapore, Trevor made it clear that it did not appeal to him, so that was that. The following year Ross too was nominated for interview, but like Trevor was hesitant and did not pursue it.

Jennifer has always been very diligent and creative. In fact when in pre-school, her teacher told us that a visiting state director had been impressed by Jennifer's organisational skills in the playground, and that she said she would be interested in following her through the years; rather like the Seven Up series. Had she done so, she would be truly amazed at Jennifer's capabilities. She has always downgraded her abilities and although she was well above average in the highest stream, she felt overshadowed by the boys, I am sure. Always conscientious with her schoolwork, one occasion stands out in my mind when she was about seven. She was doing her homework finishing off drawings to complement her written work, which was to be displayed on the classroom wall during a visit by a school inspector. Her teacher had stressed the importance of the displays for the inspector, which just shows how we can mislead children in the pursuit of excellence. Jennifer's drawing showed many hats in a shop window, no doubt inspired by shopping with her mother. After labouring for hours decorating the different hats, she was distraught at not being able to come up with fresh ideas for the last two hats. I had to persuade her that the inspector would not have time, nor would she notice such detail amongst all the other children's work.

Even as a child in primary school, she was very inventive, coming up with extraordinary ideas for costumes for book-week celebrations. One year she simply put a brown quilted saucer chair cover (these cane chairs were popular in the sixties) over her back, and with black stockings on legs and arms she crouched down on all fours and crawled slowly across the stage. It was a fine portrayal of the tortoise in The Hare and the Tortoise. The following year she added black spots and again with black stockings walked in the parade as The Magic Pudding (the spots resembling currants in the pudding). Incidentally, she won first prize on both occasions. This inventiveness is shown in everything she does to this day, whether it be designing fancy dress costumes from bits and pieces, making toys, creating gifts and greeting cards, cooking or sewing. She claims the best gift she ever received was her sewing machine, which Errol gave her in her teens. Her most cherished gift is a star sapphire, which we brought back from India in the mid-eighties. Now the 7th July 2002, I have just given her my engagement and eternity rings, as I can longer wear them as they slip off my hand. With touching emotion, she declared she would value them forever, as part of both Errol and me.

Although she has continued with a desire for perfection in her work, as an Education Officer with the Tasmanian Parks and Wildlife she has learned to discriminate between the important and unimportant detail. She is very quick with all she tackles and her energy is boundless. Consequently, she achieves an incredible amount in one day and it is hard to keep up with her.

Aside from all the above, we have a few endearing memories. She and I were about to fly to Adelaide to see my mother, who was in a nursing home. Before leaving home, I asked how I looked, to which she replied at age four, 'Mummy you look devising.' From an early age whenever we drove past the APPM factory on the Burnie foreshore, she always started the chorus 'Block your noses!', as the smell of the factory smoke was most unpleasant.

When Errol first joined ATP (Australian Tioxide Products), he had a very dour older secretary. Even after two years, whenever I rang Errol at the office she persisted in asking who was speaking, to which I was always tempted to reply, his mistress. He was delighted when she was replaced by the very competent, young and attractive Carol Greenhill, who had a good sense of humour. He joked a lot with Carol and when he arrived home after work he sometimes said in fun to Jennifer, when she kissed and hugged him, 'Come on, you can do better than that. Carol gives me better kisses.' One day Jennifer and I were returning from Ulverstone, and stopped to buy a drink at a shop in Sulphur Creek. Behind the counter was Errol's former secretary who addressed me by name. Later Jennifer asked who the lady was, and on being told that she was Daddy's secretary before Carol, Jennifer aged four sniffed, 'Not much good for kissing.' To this day twenty-two years after Errol's termination with ATP, (Carol resigned in support of him), we still keep in touch with her and husband Lance. Each year Errol phones Carol, or she him, on Secretary's Day.

A story comes to mind. We were driving in Melbourne when a car suddenly cut across in front of us. The boys then aged three and two, instantly stood up in the in the back, banged on our seats, and cried out in unison 'Bugger, Bugger, Bugger!' It was obvious where they learned that.

Although Errol has a passion for dogs and can never see one without whistling to it, we have never had a dog. I once declared that if Errol got me pregnant, I would produce pups. In Burnie, all the neighbours' dogs did their business on our lawns so we got sick of cleaning it up, especially with our young children around. Trevor once pleaded for a little dog, which would do tiny poohs, but to no avail.

One evening when they were quite small, there was a sound and movement at the back door, which the boys said must be a spook. On investigation, we found a female tabby cat, which they immediately christened Spooky and declared that they wanted to keep. Despite Errol's protest that he was allergic to cat's fur, Spooky became a much-loved part of our family for eighteen years. (It was on Jennifer's fifth or sixth birthday that he agreed she could stay.) He insisted she stay outside but of course she ventured inside, encouraged by the children, including the time she gave birth to her litter of two in the comfort of the linen cupboard and then lay with them on the sofa bed in the sunroom. One evening Errol came home and found them all sunning themselves on the sofa, and was most upset at our lack of consideration because of his allergy. He was surprised to learn that they had been lying there for some weeks as had Spooky before, over which time he had never sneezed or had his eyes swell; nor did he during the next eighteen years. We kept one female tabby kitten, named simply Tabby, who had a long, happy life extending over seventeen years. The black male kitten was adopted by a friend, but within a few days met a sad fate under a wheel of their car. Both Spooky and Tabby when elderly, endured the plane trip to Sydney where they slowly adjusted to their new home, Spooky better than Tabby, who was always very nervous. Spooky, I believe suffered a heart attack, and was buried in our garden by a tearful Errol and Ross, and Tabby was put to sleep by the vet. In hindsight, it may have been kinder to leave them with neighbours in Burnie, as both cats were frequent and welcome visitors to their homes, as I learned on the verge of leaving.

When pregnant with Petrina I attended an evening pottery class held in the old Parklands High School buildings down on the foreshore near Burnie Park. It was a fun class held in a room under the recently vacated school and under the experienced tuition of Geoff Makin, who had recently arrived from England. I was more enthused about this craft and a couple of years later enrolled in a new ceramics certificate course, which was due to commence the following year.

However, following the disastrous February fires in Hobart in 1967, kilns and equipment intended for Burnie were directed to schools that had suffered fire damage. As they expected the ceramics course was to be postponed for only a few months, it was suggested that I start the Art Certificate with painting and drawing, which I did. The ceramics was postponed indefinitely, so I continued with art and finally after four years had a piece of paper to show for my efforts. While studying painting and drawing for many years I had never had any qualifications. In my third year, I met a girl, who was teaching art at Burnie High, and as she was pregnant was resigning. Wendy suggested that I apply for the part-time position, which was four-fifths of a full load. I had no teaching experience and was very hesitant, but Peggy Gill convinced me to try, as she had no teaching qualifications or experience when she started as a commerce teacher.

My teaching career

I was interviewed by the North-West Superintendent of Schools, Ray somebody, who was most encouraging. In fact, I overheard his phone conversation with his superior in Hobart, when he claimed that I was a highly intelligent woman. This comment amused me, as Ray barely knew me and had probably made the assumption based on my being the wife of a man with position in the community. An interview followed with the principal, who was against employing me without teaching experience. In fact, he was against me for the next eight years of his term as principal, and thwarted me in every way as he was want to do with staff and students alike. At the close of one year, the departing students paraded a pig's head, mounted on a car with a suitable placard declaring their pleasure at leaving the school. 'Pig' was what they called him. My interview with the very young head of the Art Department, Alan Turner, was entirely different. Alan, recently returned from St Martin's School of Art in London (a place I had studied), was a recipient of one of the first Churchill Fellowships offered. He was much more supportive and talked me into trying it.

So, aged forty-three my teaching career commenced. At the end of my first year, I was given the option of continuing on a full time basis and went on to teach for a further ten years. I loved it so much and could not believe that I was being paid, especially during term vacations and the six weeks Christmas break. As it was, I was spending so much extra time preparing lessons and cleaning up the art room that I opted for full time. It proved ideal, as I was still home in time for the children after school and able to spend the school holidays with them as well.

From the time Ross started school, he and Trevor walked up the steep hill home. On occasions Trevor went home with Peter Burrell, and later with Leslie Simpson when he moved to Burnie. Our Trevor Leslie was delighted to find that they shared a name. Ross often went home with Garry Collins whose family lived above their baker's shop opposite the school. After such a visit a happy Ross returned home with his navy, school uniform covered with flour. In turn, Jennifer joined the boys walking home with Jenny Wood, and Kim and Roxanne Proverbs. They enjoyed the walk even in the north-west coastal rain, when they would appear at the back door like little drowned rats in bright yellow raincoats. Those were the days when children were not spoiled, besides there was no choice for I had no car then, nor was there a bus. Sometimes Errol went to work with another member of staff until he was supplied with a car a few years on. As his cars were updated, I inherited a couple of Valiants that he had used first.

Jennifer studied ballet well into her teens, under the tuition of the well-qualified Miss Winsome Stalker. She went on the way home from school and I collected her at the end of class. I do not know how often it happened but I shudder to think that a caring mother could forget to pick up her daughter even once, leaving her waiting in the cold as I did. That is one memory that still haunts me all these years later. In spite of this neglect, Jennifer loved her ballet and performed in many concerts in Burnie and Devonport. It is interesting to note that the famous Australian dancer and choreographer, Graeme Murphy, studied in Launceston and possibly attended some productions. On our return from our family visit to London, where Jennifer and I were lucky enough to get tickets to see Rudolph Nureyev, Jennifer would not tell Miss Stalker that we had seen him dance at Covent Garden because everyone would think she was spoilt and boasting. None of the children told anyone of their pending overseas trip, for exactly the same reason.

The year after I started teaching, Trevor entered Burnie High, and I drove him and his friend Gary Fielding to and from school. Invariably I was running late in the mornings and as I manoeuvred our VG Valiant down Bay Street, the boys taunted me with the old nickname of 'Jack Brabham'. Although a mere ten-minute drive, I was often a few minutes late and the eagle eyes of Mr Paul Rollins were always watching for me from his window. Many other teachers were late but they were smarter than I was, and parked up on the hill behind the school - a spot of which I was unaware. The senior mathematics teacher, who lived nearby and walked to school, was notorious for being half an hour late. He was even late for class and students reported that he used to disappear during lessons to check on the building of his new home.

I got on well with the art staff. Kit Hiller was a brilliant young artist in all media and went on to a celebrated career. Her work has been shown in the Archibald Portrait Prize and she has won the Portia Geach prize for female artists twice. The fourth member, Nigel Lazenby, assisted me in creating three dimensional mixed media paintings using plaster, string and inks, for which I was awarded a credit in my final assessment. Nigel left to freelance and is also most successful. His replacement was first year teacher, Stephen Rainbird, a clever young man, who very soon became disenchanted with the limitations of teaching and moved on to gallery directing. He is currently Curator of the University of Queensland Art Gallery. Despite the twenty year difference in age, he preferred the company of the older women in our staff room to the younger staff, as had Nigel before him. We all had lots of fun and became very good friends. To this day we still hear from Steve every Christmas, and I correspond regularly with Shirley Robinson and occasionally with Fay Croome - my two special friends from Burnie High days. Shirley is wonderful in keeping me up to date with Burnie news and sends cuttings of the vibrant local art scene, and any mention of old associates.

A year after I started teaching, Alan Turner, only twenty-eight years old, was tragically killed when he was run off the road by a car travelling on the wrong side. The driver of the other car, an American, was unhurt. Unfortunately, even Alan's Jaguar did not save him.

While teaching part-time I was still trying to keep up my social commitments, and was more than happy to give these up when offered full time work. After all, we were still busy with evening engagements and entertaining in our home. Anyone, who thinks life in a country town is boring, has probably not experienced it for themselves. In regional centres like Burnie, where distance and traffic are not an issue, there often still are excellent restaurants and sporting venues, uncrowded beaches, local entertainment and occasionally visiting shows. When one considers that one can drive the length of the state from Launceston to Hobart, in the same time as a round trip from our Sydney suburb of Turramurra to Bondi on a Saturday night, it is far easier to go out of one's way on special occasions.

After driving home from school, I have happy memories of sitting in the car chatting with Trevor, which we both enjoyed. In his pre-school years, Trevor would sit with me while I was entertaining women friends in the sunroom. Later, after they had left, he commented that he liked listening to our conversation, as 'You can learn a lot Mummy' - how wise he was! Truly, out of the mouth of babes.

In his first year at high school, I taught Trevor's class, all of whom were in the top stream, Level III. They soon dispelled the much-quoted notion that science and maths inclined students are not artistic. This misguided assumption, to my mind, is based on the fact that the academic student is often forced to specialise and to choose between science and arts. They were a pleasure to teach, as not only were they keen, but instinctively recognised the principles of design and colour.

One student, Theresa Campbell, claimed that I might be favouring Trevor in his marks, so I suggested that the students themselves should compare and honestly assess the class' work together, which they did. Surprise, surprise, they came up with my assessment for each student, placing Trevor in the top ten with a high pass, which placated Theresa. Everyone was happy, including me.

I taught Jennifer for one year, but not Ross. Both Trevor and Jennifer were more interested in art at school, though Ross always had a fine appreciation - especially in later years. Jennifer enrolled in HSC and has since joined pottery classes. Very recently, she completed a competent first attempt pastel drawing of apples on a Mother's Day card for me. While still at high school, Trevor, together with his friend Trevor Leonard, somehow managed to attend an adult life drawing class at the technical college! Trevor Leonard was always very accomplished and is now teaching art in Launceston. At the end of Year 8, Trevor was heartbroken when he had to give up technical subjects such as woodwork and architectural drawing. This is a common problem for students with wide interests; even more so for those pursuing science and mathematics subjects that often have pre-requisite subjects. I don't recall any such dilemma with Ross, who was not inclined to talk about his concerns, nor even worry before exams. Trevor, before setting off to sit his first HSC exam asked could he have a small brandy to settle his stomach. Later his Chemistry teacher asked whether Trevor was happy with the paper, and when I relayed the above incident he was surprised that Trevor should be nervous. As he knew everything what was there to be nervous about? By contrast, before his first HSC exam, I asked Ross if he was nervous, to which he jokingly replied, 'Can't you see? I'm shaking all over.' He was perfectly relaxed, adding that he never got nervous.

In those days in Tasmania, HSC students who were doing the advanced science subjects (Physics, Chemistry) were required to spread the units over two years. Other matriculating subjects were examined after one year of study, and thus it was possible for some students to matriculate and enter university when they were only sixteen. The vast majority, like Trevor and Ross were a year older. Both boys were named in the top twenty students at the end of their HSC. As well, the Professor of Chemistry at university asked Ross what mark he had received, and on being told commented that he remembered it well, as it was the highest result he had ever given!

Our children grow up

Both boys wanted a career in science and on the advice of our friend, Dr Geoff Haward, Head of Education Launceston TCAE, they accepted teaching scholarships, which were available at that time. The scholarships paid them throughout their four years at university, after which they were obliged to teach for two years, or repay the money. The boys were particularly attracted to this scheme, which gave them some independence, as they thought they should be by the age of seventeen. The alternative was for us to keep them for four years, living away from home in Hobart. We did not object to doing this but they preferred otherwise.

In hindsight this may have been a retrograde decision, as teaching and a general science degree do not always offer as much, no matter how good the results. As they would have been accepted into any professional degree; medicine, law or engineering may have rewarded them more. Although they enjoyed teaching, there was insufficient challenge and not much recognition for initiative within the public school system. At a time when leave without pay was encouraged, both travelled overseas.

Trevor went for a year to Europe via India and Nepal. He had previously travelled, immediately after university for six weeks in Papua New Guinea, spending some time living with the highland tribesmen in their huts. Lisa Cuatt, a friend of Jennifer's, had accompanied him and it was a great experience for them both.

A year later, Trevor aged twenty-four had been accepted into medicine at Flinders University, Adelaide, and the University of NSW. As he wanted a break before embarking on another five years of study, he decided to defer medicine and to travel for a year. He cut his travel a little short, however, and although we knew that he had not been well, he arrived home unexpectedly. By then we were living in Sydney, and one Saturday we were just about to go to tennis when we saw someone wearing a small backpack casually coming down our driveway. It was our prodigal son looking in every way as though he was returning from a day's outing, not a year of travel overseas. Being very practical he had been determined not carry too much, and had chosen a very light pack and discarded all non-essentials. On his return he was not at all well, and in addition to amoebic dysentery, seemed to have contracted some form of chronic fatigue. His symptoms were insomnia, exhaustion, panic attacks, sweating and loss of weight for two years and to a lesser degree for years thereafter. Although he went to Adelaide, he abandoned the idea of studying medicine, returning to Tasmania and teaching.

After teaching for two and half years, Ross too had itchy feet and headed for Thailand and then onto London. He taught intermittently in the East End of London, and combined work with further travel throughout Europe. On his return a couple of years later, he met up with Trevor (then on long service leave) in Los Angeles and they travelled together around the US and into Canada.

Ross, on his return to Australia, taught for a year before starting a postgraduate course at the University of Tasmania in Hobart. He was offered a very nice redundancy, due to a cutback in staff, after teaching for only two years! He then moved onto Melbourne, and then Canberra where he has been working as a government patent examiner for the last twelve or so years.

On the other hand Trevor had held out for years in the hope of a redundancy, but was considered too valuable to let go as had been teaching Physics, Maths and later Information Technology for much of his teaching life at Launceston College. In the end, he was despairing of the many changes to the system and the degradation of teaching quality in his disciplines. He was genuinely concerned about the students and their education, and kept saying, 'Who will teach them if I leave?' However, he was given little choice, when as part of statewide cuts he was transferred to Campbell Town District High School. No one else would accept the position, as it involved staying overnight or a long round trip each day; Trevor being unmarried was an easy choice. He was teaching grades at a level far below his qualifications. The students were largely unruly and defiant, and he often joked that his subjects were now self-esteem and discipline. With no opportunity to join the state Public Service transfer list, he resigned.

After briefly working for the Launceston City Council on geographic information systems, he came to Sydney and joined Errol in working for a small company. They were importing scientific instruments and aircraft equipment among other things. Three years later, he moved to Melbourne to work as a business consultant for a further three years, and is currently the Australian representative for a Singaporean IT company.

I have raced ahead of myself. As the French say, 'Retournons a nos moutons', or, 'Let us return to our sheep'; in this case to the seventies, and my teaching career and life in Burnie.

Returning to study

In the mid-seventies, staff that did not hold a Tasmanian Teachers Certificate were told it would become a necessary qualification for all teachers. The only State to have a professional certificate at the time, it was awarded after teacher training and one or two years actual teaching. At a minimum, it would involve study and assignments in three education subjects: Principles and Practices of Teaching, Psychology and Philosophy. Three of us in our forties, Fay Croome, Rhoda Turner, and I, embarked on this course with great trepidation. Two nights a week we were tutored from 5 to 6 p.m., before which I rushed home from school to ensure dinner was all prepared. Fortunately, distances between venues were short and I became a master at preparing meals in advance. Actually, I think I thrived on it as have always loved a challenge and studying.

Every month or so we had assignments based on our particular area of teaching. These required much research, which I found particularly interesting and stimulating in the field of art. At these times, I sat up until the early hours night-after-night, often as late as four a.m. My one problem was keeping within the word limit, as we were penalised for not doing so. Carol, Errol's capable secretary was a godsend as she typed the finished assignments before mailing to Hobart for assessment. No matter how scribbled or the number of insertions I had, Carol interpreted my thoughts with perfect accuracy. After presenting our first assignment, all three of us, Fay, Rhoda and I were certain of failure and waited with apprehension for the results. When Fay came into our staff room chortling she had received an 'A' for her efforts, as had Rhoda, I thought her very inconsiderate. I would surely be embarrassed when forced to disclose my result. Imagine my joy on finding in the mail that I too had been awarded an 'A'. The other younger and more confident teachers received much lower results. We three did not rest on our laurels, as we felt it would be difficult to maintain the same grade; and so put even more effort into subsequent assignments. However, we continued to receive A grades and gained High Distinctions at the end of the year. I could not bear the thought of two more years of study and decided to tackle the remaining two subjects in the following year. They proved to be less intense and again I passed with flying colours and Distinctions. Despite my success, Mr Rollins refused to give his seal of approval for my TTC until the following year, when Fay and Rhoda completed their studies. This in turn affected my classification depriving me of a salary increase for that year.

Our children spent all of their growing up years in Tasmania, over which time they developed a great love for the state - as Errol and I have too. Regardless of where they have since travelled or lived, they still think of it as home. It is surprising how many Taswegians have a curiosity about the rest of the world, travelling for extensive periods but invariably returning to roost.

Friends in Tasmania

Over those eighteen years, Errol and I enjoyed our life in Burnie and made many lifelong friends, including Joan and Royce Neville (until their deaths), and especially Peggy and David Gill. Peggy, sadly, has Alzheimers and is in a home in Hobart, but David whom we see occasionally is still very young and active. Other early friends such as the Minns divorced after their return to England and then remarried! Dear Derek died aged only fifty-three and Margaret, Jennifer's devout godmother, who remembered every birthday and Christmas her entire life, died in her early sixties. We were reunited a few times, the last time when Margaret and her second husband stayed with us in Sydney on a trip to Australia. Jennifer also made the long train trip from Holland to visit her while they were living near Malaga in Spain. Ailee and Roy Lauder moved to Burnie when Roy was appointed Superintendent of North-West General Hospital, and we spent many hours over dinner and playing bridge in their company. Both Ailee and Roy were excellent cooks, and we were sorry to leave them when we moved to Sydney. Although she was much younger, I had a special rapport with Pam de Bomford, whom I met when she and her family moved opposite us on Seaview Avenue. Jennifer and Johnnie played together, and were mothered by his sweet and caring older sister Louise. Phyl and Geoff Haward transferred to Launceston, and have remained our good friends to this day. They entertained us many times in their home and at Hawley Beach, a delightful little known hideaway near Devonport. They later up-dated this beach shack to become their home for retirement. They keep in touch when passing through Sydney and we try to see them when we are in Tasmania.

Rita Simpson

My very dearest friend was Rita Simpson, who had a very sad life, and despite all remained cheerful and ever optimistic. Although Trevor and Leslie were friends, as were Carol and Ross, I did not really know Rita well until Ross and Carol performed together in a school play. We were soul mates and from then on became bosom friends. She was the loveliest person I have ever known and I can honestly say the only friend I have truly loved. Her life was cut short in her early fifties, when after a year of suffering she died of stomach cancer. She had moved to Sydney shortly before us, to start a new and wonderful life as both her children were at university in Hobart. However she was enticed back to Burnie by her selfish ex-boss, who could not manage without her. A year later, he retired and she moved to Hobart to be near Leslie and his wife Lyn, who looked after her in her final months. I still cry when I think of her. She deserved so much better in life. As Steve Rainbird so rightly said, those of us who had known Rita were most fortunate.

My eleven years of teaching were happy. A pleasant friendship and shared interest in bridge developed with Val Mitchell. She was a teacher of mathematics and her husband Bob an engineer with Savage River Mines in the north-west. After a move to Singapore and now for many years in Perth WA, our friendship has endured.

Transfer to Parklands

After nine years at Burnie High, I was dismayed when I first heard of my transfer to Parklands High School High. I was contented where I was, particularly as we had a new principal. However, the transfer turned out to be a most enjoyable and rewarding two years for me. What a different atmosphere it was! The staff was most congenial due to the friendly and sociable principal, Noel Atkins. Each day commenced with coffee in the general staff room and no one was ever late. Morning recess gatherings were jovial occasions and not to be missed; not to mention the tasty sandwiches and scones provided by the Home Economics staff. I joined the luncheon soup club, and was forever challenged when it was my turn to prepare a soup for the other eight members. The most memorable soup was made by the bachelor vice-principal. I had never been much of a soup maker before, but my family were served some delicious soups thereafter. There were many social dinner parties when all staff gathered at Rosy Faulkner's home. Rosy was a divorcee with two small children and as senior librarian was not only capable in her job, but made herself available for anyone and anything that needed doing. She was, and still is, totally unflappable and no matter how busy still finds time for more. She truly fits the adage, 'if you want something done then ask a busy person'.

We instantly struck up a friendship, which continues today. At the time I left Burnie, she moved to Hobart, joining the staff of Hutchins school. Her many interests extended to doing flowers for school and university functions, when she would collect flowers from her own vast garden and elsewhere. Always a keen gardener she set about planting about forty rhododendrons. She had always bred cats, now numbering nineteen, many of which she sold overseas. Whenever we went to Hobart, she insisted we stay with her. When Errol and I rose one morning, we were welcomed by a choice of fish for breakfast. Rosy had risen at five a.m. and delivered a cat to the airport to be shipped to New Zealand, after which, she and a friend had gone fishing. For lunch we had freshly caught lobster, with homegrown salad and peach pie made with Rosy's preserves from the garden. Having a keen interest in art she decided to do Fine Arts majoring in pottery, and at the school, she met and married John Mitchell - also an enthusiastic potter. Even when her children were small, she was continually looking for another challenge, the next being studying for an MA to add to her list of qualifications. Now, she and John run their own gallery cum restaurant in Salamanca Place, Hobart, and yet Rosy still finds time to judge at cat shows around Australia and overseas. On our last visit, we tramped up the hill on their property at Taroona to view the tiny peacock chicks they had bred. Needless to say, each day Rosy made the trip in order to feed her small charges.

Holidays from Tasmania

Whilst in Tasmania, our holidays were in the main restricted to visiting Mum in South Australia. After a stroke she lived with Helen for at least a year, and then moved to a nursing home for a further year. It was so sad to see her like a vegetable, so thin and gaunt that I could not recognise my own lovely mother. Dad continued living at home in

Tasmania

Burra, driving to Adelaide at weekends to sit with Mum. After Mum died he too suffered the same fate, finishing up in a repatriation hospital in Adelaide. As they did with Mum, Aunties Kath and Jess took it in turns, and of course, Fuff and Helen visited constantly. It was a heavy burden for the family to carry all those years. Auntie Kath was delighted when she took Dad to her home, sat him down and reported that he sang – giving us hope. Although he seemed to be recovering, darling Dad could not bear the thought of being useless and dependent on others. I returned to Burra for his funeral, but had not made it for Mum's as Auntie Kath had just arrived in Burnie for a well-earned break. Instead we went to church and prayed. Fortunately, neither of my parents lived to witness Helen's suffering or Fuff's tragic loss when her husband Bob had a sudden heart attack, and died on Christmas Eve. Since then our visits to South Australia have been much happier occasions.

Around 1965, the Dollman family donated a bookcase for prayer books to commemorate Dad's long association as soloist and warden of the church. When the bookcase was installed, a special service was held in St Mary's, Burra to celebrate the event and the life of Donald Redding, who had recently passed away. I returned from Tasmania for the service, as did Clem Davey, who was then living in Hobart and teaching music at a high school. Clem disclosed that he had once shared a flat with a very good friend of ours, George Inglis. Later George told me that Clem was homosexual; little wonder that he was disinterested in Peg or Rae!

I have indeed been blessed in having two other mothers, Kath and Jess, until their deaths when aged ninety-seven and one-hundred-and-one years respectively. Auntie Kath visited us twice in Burnie, the last time with Uncle Lou Avery shortly after their marriage. Many times she came to Sydney accompanied by Fuff, my caring and loving elder sister.

Errol and I took an organised tour to Singapore, Thailand, Hong Kong, Taiwan and Japan. In Japan, we spent a few days soaking up the culture in each of Tokyo, Kyoto, and under winter snow in a traditional ryokan in the resort of Hakone. This trip further stimulated my interest in Japanese culture.

As well as our overseas trip with the children, we had a wonderful three-week holiday in New Zealand, taking Jennifer and Fuff. On this trip as it was vacation time, we left our sensible teenagers alone in the house, under the watchful eye of our good neighbours. On returning we were met at the airport by the sight of Ross with his arm in a sling, which we initially thought was a joke, but no, he had indeed broken his arm the day after our departure. In his usual exuberant fashion, he had run down the freshly painted steps at the back of our house (done by Errol a few days before to please me), but this time they were wet after rain and very slippery. Despite frequent contact by phone, they did not breathe a word of his mishap to us.

Errol leaves Tioxide

In 1977, Errol parted company with Tioxide, eighteen months after Dr Keith Sugars replaced Don Fraser as General Manager, a role that might have gone to Errol, who was then Commercial Manager. Sugars, appointed by the Board in England, was a very arrogant man and disliked by all staff. In spite of this and although he gave Sugars his full support, Errol baulked at the idea of his staff attending meetings at weekends, particularly after they had already worked overtime at the end of the financial year. This was just one of the many unreasonable demands Sugars placed on the staff. Sugars then plotted against Errol by, among many other things, deliberately withholding the correct commencement time for a meeting of directors. Errol arrived late, something that he would never do, as he abhors lateness.

He then joined the practice of a young accountant, to whom he trustingly lent money for enlarging his premises, which incidentally, he has never got back. Two years later, he was approached by a competitor of Tioxide's, Laporte Australia, to apply for the position of Financial Controller. He had a long-standing relationship with both the Chairman, Bill Duffield (Duffy and wife Phyl) and the Managing

Director, John Cordner (and wife Gwen). His application was successful and required a move to Sydney, which appealed to us.

Jennifer was in her final year at Hellyer College. The Higher School Certificate years of Burnie High became Hellyer College in name only, when Trevor was in Year 12, and then opened its doors at the new premises the year after. Hellyer was the first college purpose-built for community access, adult education and the HSC in Tasmania, and in fact Australia.

Sydney, New South Wales

Errol moved to Sydney in December 1979 to check out the housing situation, and to see whether the job and Sydney fulfilled his expectations. Meanwhile, Jennifer and I remained in Burnie to allow her to finish Year 12, encouraging local gossip that Errol and I had separated! Towards the end of that year, we put the house on the market, although there were few buyers in the district. In the event of not making a quick sale, I approached Mr Rollins (now District Supervisor) with the intention of resigning. To my surprise the same man, who had been anti my every move, proposed that I not burn my bridges too soon and rather than resign, to ask for three months leave commencing January 1980. He also suggested, that if I wanted, I could cancel the leave at the start of the year and so continue teaching if our house had not been sold. Brian Adams, a South African, who had bought an optometrist practice was showing genuine interest and eventually after three months made us an offer. He and his wife Marlene drove a hard bargain, and as we had by then bought a house in Sydney, we were forced to accept.

Jennifer started university at the beginning of the year and I was alone in the house until the Adams moved in. As I was obliged to teach until June, I moved into Bill Fry's home next door, which had been empty since Bill went to a nursing home. This was an ideal arrangement, for it was fully furnished, and I knew the house well as Errol and I had been looking after Bill since the death of his wife Win. We took him meals and many times picked him up from the floor after his day at the club. He was a heavy drinker, and after Win died, got through a bottle of brandy a day and a flagon of sherry a week. We have a funny story about Bill in hospital. After an operation, Bill was begging the sister for a brandy but she would only bring him water. After a few sips, he said to us, 'You know, this isn't a bad drop.' I think he had never tasted water before! He was a dear man, whom Win had blamed for their not having children. When reminiscing one day he confessed to me his deep dark secret. Despite Win's claims, he revealed that while living in Samoa (he was an agent for a shipping line), he had sired a daughter by their Samoan housemaid, a fact unknown to Win.

For eighteen months, Errol rented an apartment in McMahon's Point by the harbour. He came home once a month, at great expense, and I visited Sydney during school holidays to look for a house. This posed a great problem, as house prices rose by 40 per cent in 1979, and each house we looked at was $10,000 more but less appealing than ones we had seen the day before. We had made an offer, which was accepted, on a lovely home when Errol first went to Sydney. The day I was returning to Tasmania we heard that we been gazumped. Incidentally, a year later, this house at Northbridge on the desirable Lower North Shore had doubled in value and today will have escalated to well over one million dollars - more so than the house we bought a year later and paid more for. As we could no longer afford to buy in this area, we focused on the leafy suburbs of the Upper North Shore. We must have looked at a hundred houses before finding one that appealed and was affordable. Eventually we went to auction and again paid more than we had anticipated. We had two houses in Tasmania, our home in Burnie and a house in Sandy Bay, Hobart, which we bought when Ross joined Trevor at university. Together these contributed to only half the price of the house in Sydney. Although it is all water under the bridge now, it took years to pay off the principal together with interest. Ironically, when we bought our Burnie home eighteen years before and even the house in Hobart three years previously, there was very little difference in real estate prices between the States.

However, we have been happy here at Finlay Road, surrounded by its temperate forest, for twenty-two years now and even our offspring regard it as home. It is a large clinker brick and timber, split level house with pool and wide surrounding decking. It overlooks a creek, which runs through the property, and is set back from the street with no sound of traffic. It is hard to believe that one is in a big city and people often say they feel as though they have been transported to a peaceful island in the tropics. All is lush and green, with ground ferns and tall tree ferns intermingled with huge umbrella trees, monstera deliciosa climbing up trees, elephants ears, bamboo standing more than fifteen metres high, giant strelitzia, the flowers from which the lorikeets drink the morning dew, plus a backdrop of towering eucalypts. We have planted more natives and some flowering exotics: bougainvillea, hibiscus, camellias, agapanthus, hydrangeas and clivia to name a few, which add a touch of colour. Add to all this, the soothing sound of little waterfalls in the trickling creek, which turns into a torrent after rain. Once the waters of the creek extended at least thirty feet in width. The sound of rushing water is equally comforting and exciting. As well as the birds, we have possums clambering over the roof and decking at night, and happy frogs in our creek!

The house, which featured in House and Garden shortly before we moved in, is even more attractive I believe with the changes we have made. A kitchen cum breakfast room, dining room and front entrance hall are on the middle level. From the entrance hall, stairs lead up to three bedrooms and two bathrooms, and another few stairs lead down to the lower level and the enormous open living room, which extends the full length of the house. It is the equivalent of three rooms, and includes a small bar room. Here multiple French doors open to 60' of decking, making it ideal for entertaining. Throughout the house there are walls of full-length windows, and upstairs, doors lead from the bedrooms to a covered balcony. The main bedroom is very large, with another long room adjoining with a sink and cupboards that can be used as a dressing room and kitchen. There is a door here, which opens to the double garage below, though at present shelves holding boxes of my cards block it off. Our home is unusual in design and décor, and the setting is much admired.

Jennifer preferred to be with her brothers and friends, and to attend university in Hobart. Since the sale of our house in Sandy Bay, Trevor had moved to a delightful two-storey flat, which was once the coach-house and stable of a huge home with extensive gardens. Jennifer happily moved in with him and I joined Errol in Sydney knowing that she was in capable and caring hands. After fending for themselves since the age of seventeen, our boys were good cooks and Jennifer soon learned too. She had done domestic science at school, and Ross, who always showed a keen interest in food had done cooking too. He now is an excellent cook devising his own daring recipes.

With the three children happily settled in Hobart, a new phase of my life began. In June 1980 and approaching my fifty-fourth year, I joined Errol at 45 Finlay Road, Warrawee. (There has been some confusion over the suburb's boundary, however, as the other side of the street is in Turramurra).

Baldwin St International

We were most fortunate, as the Cordners had introduced Errol to a private tennis group, named the Baldwin Street International Tennis Club, and hosted at the home of Mary and Keith Lewis. The members numbered about thirty and originally heralded from various states, while a few were from overseas. Someone had designed a flag that was hoisted every Saturday afternoon, and we had our own song proclaiming that Keith was the President because he owned the bloody tennis court. Our club cry was, 'Balls, balls, balls to the President!' After tennis we sojourned to the rumpus room, where a few non-playing members joined the gathering for drinks, much hilarity and storytelling. Then at seven or later, we might go out to dinner or get take-away. On rainy days, we took turns in having drinks at our homes in the late afternoon. Many members had known each other for years and others were introduced by existing players. All were compatible with a common sense of humour. Many of the men from the southern states were ex-footballers and keen AFL fans, and often had to be torn away from the TV to play tennis. Incidentally, we paid no fees, but all contributed to afternoon tea, drinks, and in providing food for our Christmas parties. Mary and Keith were most generous hosts and went to no end of trouble for all occasions.

At the Christmas parties Keith, who was Sales Manager for the Royal Agricultural Society, presented all the ladies with unused sashes from the Easter Show. These presentations were accompanied by appropriate and humorous speeches. For example, prolific breeder or champion producer of milk - the latter going to a lady with an ample bosom. All members received prizes for their various talents, whether tennis or otherwise. I received a toy rabbit in reward for my attempts to chase after every ball and another year a candy pink bouffant wig, for what I do not recall. Highlights were our Elegance Dinners, the second of which was held at the home of Mary and Bill Arnold. They were truly unforgettable nights, when the spirit of bonhomie and talent of all came to the fore. Seven males each prepared one of the seven courses. One wife (only I know), did step in to save the night. Dressed to the nines in dinner suits and evening gowns, with sumptuous meal and magnificent table setting it was indeed an elegant affair. The pièce de résistance was the suckling pig. It was selected and fattened for the occasion and cooked by chefs John Cordner and Bill Arnold. They carried it in proudly, complete with the traditional apple in mouth. From start to finish, it was a gourmet experience, complete with French waitresses, the like of which not even the finest French restaurant could compete with. Entertainment too was of the highest standard, courtesy of our two professionals: Gordon Boyd, a fine baritone and TV compere of Showcase; and Red Moore, singer, comedian and all round performer. Red was a member of the famous Kiwis who entertained troops during World War II and long after in peacetime. He was a clever caricaturist, and composed many of our ditties and club songs. (He passed away a few years ago.) As well, we had hilarious skits and songs performed by the very talented non-professionals amongst us. For fear of overlooking someone I hesitate to mention names, however Patty Buckle did a one woman show-stopping performance. Suffice to say this was an evening to remember.

Some years later, we had an Elegance Dinner celebrating Christmas in July. It was at Anne and Jim MacPherson's home, with seafood and traditional Christmas dinner of two large turkeys, pudding etc. The table, decorated by yours truly in their elegant dining room, followed the festive theme. This time, Jillian Boyd through her corporate catering business, obtained the services of a professional waiter. As before, we amused ourselves with a programme of skits and songs. At the end of the night, the waiter told us that in all his working life he had never enjoyed himself so much, nor come across a group, who were so entertaining and had so much fun. Flash Burdon (Errol) was appointed official photographer and we have many wonderful reminders of these memorable nights.

I believe we all felt that these nights were special and although we continue to see each other, sadly the regular tennis days ended when Keith announced the closure of our club. Keith, a keen golfer, was out early on the course on Saturdays and as he liked to watch the football on weekends as well, it was getting too much.

In August 2002, the Lewis' held a final wake for the club, as they had sold the house and land, and the court was to be redeveloped. From all accounts, it was the best party yet, and a fun auction was held to sell off the net, roller, posts and so on. The flag was lowered during the singing of the club song, followed by the usual fanfare and reminiscing. Regrettably, I missed the event as I was in hospital.

The Club Song Sheet

The Inspirational

Bring along your week's frustrations
To the game of all the nations
Feel the joys of liberation
At Lewis' tennis court.

You will find your zest returning
For a win you're really yearning
And at last you're really burning
At a game well fought.

Sydney, New South Wales

It's no place for frolics
Volley to the bollocks
Then for fun, lobs from the sun –
They're just a pair of ageing alcoholics!

Smash it! Bash it!
Cut and slash it!
Rush the net and poach and hash it!
Everyone's an expert at it –
On Lewis' tennis court.

Jolly Tennis Weather

Jolly tennis weather
Oft tempts us to play a set
We may be slow at the base line
But you ought to see us at net!

And we'll all creak together
Our bodies all racked with pain
Ready for next week's glories
Or nursing our muscular strain.

Tennis Players All

We are tennis players all
And at Baldwin Street we call
on a Saturday afternoon to play the game.
Though Evonne and Rod we prize
We can cut them down to size –
We have internationals of note and fame.

"Tennis balls" we shout in chorus
As our President we greet
We don't wish him well for nought
Though he is a damn good sport
It's because he owns the bloody tennis court!

More language studies

Eighteen months before departing Tasmania, I joined a Japanese language class tutored by an excellent teacher. As there were only three of us attending twice weekly, we progressed quickly. Soon after my arrival in Sydney, I started in the second year of a three-year course at nearby Macquarie University. There was no degree course available then so not wanting to stop I repeated one year purely for enjoyment. At Macquarie I met Jill Buddle (later Eadie), who invited me to join a group of Australian and Japanese ladies for conversation and lunch at her unit each Friday. Occasionally we met at other places, and had many luncheon parties here at Finlay Road, sitting out on our decking beside the pool. The Japanese ladies loved the subtropical setting and the colourful, friendly lorikeets and King Parrots. Many other birds frequented our paradise, like kookaburras, whip birds, butcherbirds with a beautiful song, and bellbirds with their distinctive chiming call.

I developed lasting friendships with these Japanese ladies, meeting them again when we stayed in Kazuko Matsunaga's home on a subsequent visit to Japan. Over this period, we had many Japanese students staying in our home while they studied English. We loved them all and after fifteen years still keep in touch. Two of the girls, and their husbands, stayed at our home when on their honeymoons, and all our guests except one man are married with children. Errol and I visited Seiko in Sapporo, on the northern island of Hokkaido four years ago. We travelled all over the country for four weeks by ourselves, using the very efficient fast-train system and our travelling bible the Lonely Planet guidebook. Seiko had recently lost her husband but planned a wonderful two days for us, and treated us to a night at a resort ryokan in the nearby mountains. We visited her large home where we had a traditional meal but due to her recent loss, she considered it improper to have a man stay overnight. She had so wanted us to meet Ito-san, whom she had married later in life. We travelled by train through the undersea tunnel connecting Hokkaido to Honshu. A distance of some 54 km under the sea, it is the world's longest undersea tunnel. It is indeed an engineering feat and terrifying for some to think of all that water above. This was just one of the many unusual and long-remembered experiences, which lay ahead of us in this beautiful, hospitable country.

As there was no further Japanese course available in Sydney, I enrolled in German and French, both of which I had studied at school and the latter again in Montreal.

My locked knee

We were entertaining London directors at the Australia Tower restaurant in Sydney, and about to start eating when suddenly my knee locked. I was in agony so an ambulance had to be called. It was most embarrassing leaving our visitors and being carried out through the crowded restaurant. The ambulance men managed to get me into the elevator with great difficulty as the stretcher only just fitted!

Downstairs there was even more drama. I was booked into Hornsby Hospital the next day for an operation on my faulty knee, but the ambulance could not take me 'out of their area.' They were all set to take to me to the hospital in the city, and you can imagine the fun we would have had being booked in there at 11 p.m. and then trying to arrange a transfer to Hornsby next morning! Errol convinced them he could manage if they put me in our car rather than the waiting ambulance. Errol delivered me directly to the hospital the following morning.

Trapped in a burning car

I had a setback two years later in 1986, when I had a disastrous car accident. Driving back from the northern beaches my steering failed and my car crossed the dividing lane on Mona Vale Road at St Ives colliding head-on with another car. I remember it vividly, as I had just glanced at the clock and the time was 4:40. Suddenly I was aware of the screen shattering and exploding in front of me, exactly as one sees in a film. In that short moment, my life really did flash before me. Next thing the car was on fire and I thought, 'My God, I am going to be burned alive!'

Unbelievably, I was right outside the station of the Police Rescue Squad, who came to my aid, extinguishing the fire and extricating me from the car. Thanks to them I was in Ku-ring-gai Hospital in emergency within twenty-five minutes - I noted the wall clock said 5:05. I was fully conscious during all the needle jabbing and blood transfusions, and then underwent sixty odd X-rays, which disclosed fourteen fractures throughout my body. Incredibly though my Peugeot was a write-off and I was covered in glass from the shattered windscreen, I received no facial, head or brain damage. For this I was grateful, and when a few people said that I should take a ticket in Tatts, I said there was no need as I had already been extremely lucky. Throughout my five-week stay in hospital, I forever marvelled at the speed and ability of the body to heal - both wounds and fractures. I imagined all the little healers racing around doing their job and felt privileged to be part of the miracle of rebirth. On first meeting the physio, she said she had never seen anyone with so many fractures who had lived. After weeks of intensive physiotherapy, I was back on the tennis court in six months.

After the accident, I picked up French again with the entertaining and knowledgeable Dr Emy Batache-Watt and continued for the next twelve years. We all loved her and many students stayed with the class, as it was so stimulating. I supplemented this with French through the U3A (University of the Third Age), a worldwide organisation for over fifty-fives, that offers all manner of subjects and is tutored by volunteers with minimum fees. At the same time, for fear of losing my Japanese, I attended classes at Macquarie and then privately also until two years ago. Following a trip to Spain, I tried Spanish, but was forced to give it up when I lost my voice. For six months I attended all classes, content to just listen and write, and complete homework on the computer. It all became too difficult once I had trouble walking and I was then forced to give up outings.

Flower Cards of Australia

Before my accident, I investigated the prospect of having some of my watercolour flower paintings printed in the form of greeting cards. I had already sold some paintings to home decorating shops and local galleries. Encouraged and accompanied by Trevor, I did the rounds of printers and decided upon Rodenprint. Warwick Roden and his mother June, who had founded the company with her husband, were very enthusiastic. This small family company now has over forty employees, and has won numerous Australian awards over the years. I was most impressed by the quality of the cards when they finally came off the printing press. The first printing was an expensive business, but I was prepared to lose the money and give the cards to charity if they failed to sell. I need not have worried as I sold the twelve thousand cards within three months. I had thirty six thousand more printed, adding six more designs this time, and more in the coming years.

For sixteen years with cards loaded in the boot of my car, I travelled around Sydney visiting every newsagency, gift and Australiana shop, hospital, university bookshop and anywhere where they might sell cards. I discovered shopping centres I had not known existed. I travelled the highways and byways north, south and west of Sydney, making day trips to the Central Coast, Southern Highlands and Blue Mountains, and visiting up to twelve shops en-route. Now with twenty-nine designs, I was kept busy sorting cards, packing boxes and loading the car before departing for a day's outing. When Errol and I went away for a few days or on holidays interstate, the cards accompanied us and I soon had customers all over Australia. In 2001, Trevor designed and set up my web site, www.flowercards.com.au. The site is a work of art in itself and has received many compliments, as too have the cards in the accompanying guest book. Although card orders have been few, reading the visitor's comments has been rewarding and a lot of fun.

Holidays from Sydney

Over the years since our return to Australia, Errol had had a few trips interstate and overseas, combining work with holidays in some exotic destinations. These trips increased my desire for further travel, though once in Sydney it was a few years before we ventured further afield.

Meanwhile we had some unforgettable fun holidays closer to home, especially visiting our friends Doris and Peter Cairnes on their stud property in Dorrigo – a paradise in northern NSW. Once, with Ross the organiser and his girlfriend Cheryl, we encountered a tremendous storm while celebrating my birthday on a houseboat on the lakes near Malacoota in north-eastern Victoria.

We travelled to Adelaide by various routes and one in particular stands out. With Jennifer and Ross, we went via Wilcannia where we delved into my Dad's past. We went to the hospital to talk to an old lady, who knew him well, to the school where Mum had taught for a year, and to the cemetery to find the grave of Dad's youngest sister, Ruth Dollman, who had died at the age of four. This was followed by much frustration, swearing and hilarity, when the keys were locked in the car. The cemetery was some miles out of town, and Jennifer and I set off in high spirits for help. Once on the road we were soon picked up by a truck driver, who offered to give us a lift to the local garage, but via his home first. In the meantime, Errol and Ross had succeeded in opening the car and were searching for us around the town. Needless to say, he, who shall not be named, was not amused at the delay on the long journey ahead.

We proceeded to Broken Hill where my mother had grown up, and started trawling into the past again. We found the Bryant family home on the edge of town, and I recalled my mother telling me of the nearby Afghan camps and the infamous Broken Hill two-day war at the start of World War I. Much exaggerated at the time, shots were fired when two men held up a train returning from a Sunday School picnic at Silverton. My details are sketchy but there was a short film made in which Auntie Kath was interviewed. She also attended the premiere.

Then it was on to Wilcannia where Dad, Peg and Fuff were all born, and via Wilpena Pound to the remote and vast property Oulnina Park, which was owned by the family of Errol's brother Ivor. We got a chance to experience life on a big station in the outback, and the children returned during their summer vacations to assist at the busy shearing time. Peter Burdon (Ivor's son), and his former wife Marlis, welcomed us all with wonderful meals and showed us over the extensive property. From there we went south to Adelaide passing through Orroroo, where Errol had lived for a time as a child, and Burra, where we both had lived. At each town we retraced our lives, visiting homes and schools and our favourite haunts - all of great interest to Ross and Jennifer.

Other trips include one with Jennifer to Coonabarabran, where we stayed in an old tram and walked in the area. We took advantage of a couple of short package deals: one year over Christmas to Alice Springs, Uluru, Darwin and Kakadu, and another to the beautiful Bay of Islands of New Zealand. I must not overlook, undoubtedly the most beautiful island in the world, Bali, where we spent ten days and wanted to spend the rest of our lives. We stayed first at Sanur Beach and then Ubud, the craft centre. The sheer beauty of the country, rice paddies on sloping hillsides, lovely people, exquisite food and unchanged culture, all so unspoiled overwhelmed us. Errol had been trying to get me there for many years, as he had stopped off on a business trip, but I was too pig-headed believing that it was haven for druggies. How wrong I was. Sadly, much later all this was to change on 12th October 2002, when terrorists attacked this peaceful paradise by exploding a bomb in a Kuta Beach nightclub. The results were devastating with much loss of life, and a residual fear of further terrorism among the gentle Balinese people and potential tourists.

We returned to Tasmania many times, staying once with Ross on a farm near Cressy where he did his first year of teaching. We had holidays with Trevor in his interesting old home, where he uncovered convict bricks in the fireplaces. I loved our stays at 10 Hill Street, with a magnificent view high over Launceston and only minutes away from the city. It is a perfect location, as the house is bathed in morning sun and at night has a fine view of the city lights. Trevor spent many happy hours (with some help from Errol and me), restoring the house and maintaining the garden. Although he still owns it, he has not lived there for years. Since being rented, sadly, it has fallen into a state of disrepair. I loved pottering around the garden and house - so reminiscent of my childhood home. For me and I think for Errol, perhaps of all our holidays these spent with our children have been the happiest. For the past ten years Jennifer has worked painstakingly improving her sunny home, also with a view, but of Hobart and the Derwent River.

Flinders Island

Jennifer spent her first two years of teaching on Flinders Island, which we visited in May. We were amazed by the proliferation of wildlife and especially the bird sanctuary, which was the work of an elderly colourful character, Derek Smith. He befriended Jennifer and she assisted him with banding the various species. We also met three of the most interesting personalities one could wish to meet. One a mother of five, had the most magnificent museum of stones and gemstones, all cut and polished by her from stones collected on numerous trips around Australia. Also in her museum were hundreds of old foreign bottles and coins, foraged on diving excursions from the many shipwrecks around the island. It was a museum fit to grace any large city. Next to the museum were hot houses filled with ferns and tropical plants, which she had propagated. Another surprise awaited outside, where we found a huge park of lawns with fully grown exotic and tropical trees, the like of which one would not expect to find on a windswept Bass Strait island. The most amazing thing was that all were grown from seed, gathered on her trips to warmer climes. The avenue of ten-metre high flowering gums, lining the driveway, were grown from nuts sown when she married and first moved to this sheep farm. In winter when the seas were too wild for diving, she was employed as a house painter - from the deep seas to high on a ladder!

Another lady, quite elderly and extroverted lived alone in her home. It comprised of three separate buildings in the bush, one was her bedroom, one the toilet and he third a lounge and kitchen where she greeted us. She was baking in her wood-fired oven, from which she served fresh bread with homemade berry jam. She was educated and quite charming, as was the atmosphere in spite of the dirt floor. The room was warm and inviting, with three jars of fresh flowers on the windowsill. There was a caravan for visitors, often used by people she had met while staying in New Zealand youth hostels. She was not short of money, but was frugal, ordering all basic food ingredients in bulk from Launceston. It seemed a happy sort of Robinson Crusoe existence.

The third lady had a most beautiful garden of roses, azaleas, camellias and hibiscus to mention just a few, all grown from cuttings or seed. It was every bit like a nursery with cuttings and small plants in pots, growing for her own pleasure.

Although it was May, the days were surprisingly warm. We toured the island from end to end, even including nude bathing (at Jennifer's insistence) at the deserted Chinamans Beach. On our visit to the school, we were very proud, and most impressed by Jennifer's dedication and skill in handling her combined class of kindergarten and Grade I students. Her pupils loved her and she them. On more recent visits, she has found some now married with children. She left her mark on the island by planting trees on the foreshore and assisting with other environmental endeavours.

During this time, she went to India, staying in an ashram in Delhi and then south to Pondicherry to assist with a tree-planting project, run by her friend Josh.

A QUALITY LIFE

Two years later in 1989, at the age of twenty-six, she set off all alone for Europe via Thailand. This worried us no end, especially on hearing that she arrived in Bangkok at one a.m. to find her first hotel. However she managed to enjoy her stay, and continued on to Scandinavia for the beginning of an exciting adventure that was to last for the next three years. The first of these was spent in the wilds of Sweden, assisting with the tracking and tagging of bears from a helicopter. Thence in a small boat off the northern coast of Norway with a Finnish girl, who was doing her PhD on whales. This led to volunteer work at the newly opened Whale Research Centre at Andennes, Norway and a further three northern summers of paid work. During this time she escorted a few notables, including the Duke of Edinburgh as Patron of the World Wildlife Fund.

During the northern winters, she first worked as an au pair in the ski resort of Meribel in France and then travelled to Turkey where she met Auntie Kath in Gallipoli on the seventy-fifth anniversary of the Allied defeat there. Another was spent in London and then in Whistler, Canada at a ski resort, where besides working in a pizza parlour she was able to advance her skiing skills. From there she met with friends from Meribel days and travelled down the west coast of the USA. She has kept in contact with all of these friends wherever they are in the world. Last year she worked in the Queen Charlotte Island National Park, Canada, before travelling to Alaska and thence to Sweden and Geneva for reunions with some of these northern friends. On the way home, she managed to fit in Jerusalem, Cairo, and scuba diving with her cousin Catherine in the Red Sea!

She has done many other fascinating things since, the last being environmental interpretation for a NZ company running subantarctic cruises on a chartered Russian ship. She celebrated her fortieth birthday and Christmas 2001 on the trip. January 2003, she leaves for a four-week cruise to Antarctica and is very excited. Even more so, as she has been granted a scholarship that will cover 75 per cent of the twenty thousand dollar fare.

Resuming my personal story, Errol retired from Laporte in 1985 and consulted to a large insurance broking company in North Sydney for some years. He has been most fortunate in satisfying his need to work, managing several days a week since with smaller companies. All have been pursued with amazing zest, considering that he turned eighty yesterday, on Father's Day, 1st September 2002.

Round the world - Egypt, Europe and North America

On 9th April 1988, we embarked upon a long awaited three-month tour to Egypt, Europe and North America, and then stopped off in Hawaii on our way home. We did our own thing, booking only the first few nights in Cairo before travelling by train to Luxor. We stayed at the Winter Hotel as Auntie Kath had done during the First World War, and then on to Aswan by taxi and the old majestic Cataract Gorge Hotel. We flew south to Abu Simbel to view the Aswan Dam and to see the mammoth ancient statues of Ramses the Second. The statues were relocated to higher ground last century, to save them when the valley behind the dam was flooded. The latter were truly awesome in the true sense, (to use that much overused word applied to athletes and almost anything today). We returned to Cairo where we did more of the usual tourist sights, and so much more. On Ross' recommendation we included the fascinating Tuesday camel auction, where there were hundreds of smelly noisy camels and an equal number of yelling Egyptians. The mosques were all majestic and surprisingly different in architecture. We visited the Old City, where poor families were actually living inside the ancient tombs and around the overgrown graveyard - a spine-chilling sight. As is more usual we saw the Cheops Grand Pyramid, and the stepped pyramid and tomb of sacred bulls at Saqqara.

From Cairo we flew to Amsterdam, where we picked up a hire car from the airport. For us the highlight of Holland was a visit to the famed Keukenhof Gardens, the most incredibly beautiful garden one could ever imagine. We were so lucky, as it was at the peak of spring blooming with tulips, hyacinths, daffodils, and trees in blossom everywhere.

From Holland, our trip took us through Germany, Switzerland, Austria, Italy and France, finding accommodation as we went either from the tourist information centres or by referring to our guidebook Europe on $25 a Day - a trifle out-dated! Our friends, the Phillips, who had spent a year travelling around Europe recommended places to visit and overnight stays. In France we followed a route described in my French textbook, where each chapter covered different towns and their local sights and festivals. This proved a great success, directing us to places that we would not have visited otherwise.

We crossed the Channel to England in our Peugeot hire car. We first stayed with Margaret and Tony Archdeacon (ex-Baldwin Street Tennis Club), in their lovely home in Sidcup near the city of Exeter, where John and Gwen Cordner joined us. We wined and dined at a village teahouse, and will never forget the scones and jam, and huge dish piled high with real clotted cream. While touring the Devon district we found many first-class restaurants. We then motored north to Betty and Peter Howarth, ex British Titan Products, for a repeat of hospitality extraordinaire, comprising a drive through the Lakes District, gourmet meals a la Betty and after-dinner bridge. It was then back to London to the home of my cousin Cynthia, for another lovely reunion and a drive to St Albans to revive happy memories. We also caught up with Gwen and James Halsey, while James was working in London for a time.

We returned to Paris, dropped off the car and took a flight to New York to have a few days with Midge and Norm Bentley. We hired a car to return to Montreal and see old friends, and thence to Detroit to stay with Yolan (nee Gregor) and husband Don Karcher. The next stop was Las Vegas and an aerial tour by light plane over the Grand Canyon. We saw Wendy and Malcolm Ferrier in San Diego before the final leg of our journey home. We made a stop in Hawaii and took another memorable flight - over these beautiful islands. While we had covered many miles on this trip, and viewed many magnificent sights, above all we were delighted to find all our friends in good health.

In the years since we have visited many ancient countries, soaking up the culture, and by travelling independently have met the people and experimented with the language; India, Turkey, China, Japan and Europe including our last trip to the Czech Republic, Slovakia, Hungary and Austria. We have indeed been most fortunate.

~o~

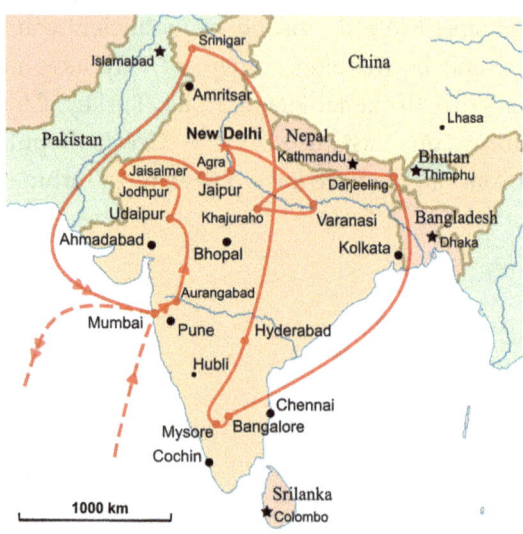

Exploring the sub-continent – our India trip

Although it is hard to choose, for me as a traveller India was the most interesting and exotic, with its fascinating history, colourful culture, magnificent palaces and past opulence – much of which has been left to decay since the British left in the forties. Despite the dreadful poverty and severely handicapped beggars, all were happy and smiling, accepting of their lot in life through religious beliefs or the continuing caste system. Even in atrocious living conditions, women were dressed in incredibly beautiful saris, a myriad of colour amongst the poverty. I will never forget the sight, in the middle of a desert, of a group of women dressed in saris of every imaginable colour, walking to the water hole with their highly polished copper pots elegantly balanced on their heads. It was like a scene out of a movie set in the desert.

Encouraged and inspired by Trevor to be independent, this was our introduction to the Lonely Planet guides, one of the first published by the enterprising couple that started the company. We planned a vague route, bought a domestic open-air ticket, made accommodation bookings for our first night in Bombay, and stays at the Lake Palace in

Udaipur (well-known from the James Bond movie Octopussy) and Rumbagh Palace Jaipur, where a Maharaja still resided. In 1986 these hotels were still quite cheap, though most luxurious.

We were awestruck by the hundred or more caves at Ellora and Ajunta in Aurangabad, north of Bombay, finding them even more impressive than any wonder of the world, including the Pyramids and Taj Mahal! Here there are ancient man-made caves with mammoth shrines and monasteries inside them. One is larger than the Parthenon and all are chiselled by hand from the ground up within the cliff face.

Everywhere we went we were dazzled by something: by colour, by gemstones, by ornate architecture, by unique clothing, detailed tapestries, handmade carpets and the mirrors of Rajasthan. We were amazed and shocked by the crude depictions of sexual intercourse between humans and beasts in extraordinary positions on fertility shrines at Khajuraho. We were horrified by the cremations at dawn on the banks of the Ganges at Varanasi (the religious centre of India), and the possibility of an odd body part floating by pilgrims bathing in the filthy water. We were charmed by the mystic atmosphere of Kashmir, the gentleness of the Muslim people, and the beauty of life on a houseboat on Dahl Lake in Srinigar, where we were treated like royalty with our own personal manservant - much as it was in the days of the Empire.

The last leg of our journey was to the top of the world, to Darjeeling. The little toy train wound up the mountainside in a corkscrew of tunnels, crossing the narrow road forty times. The township, surrounded by mountains, had deteriorated since the handover by the British in the forties. Dilapidated houses clung to the steep terraced slopes and were sadly in need of paint. The small roads and lanes were hard to negotiate, by foot or vehicle. Our Hotel Windermere, set high on the pinnacle over the town, had a magical misty view through tall fir trees to the mountains beyond. It was highly recommended by Lonely Planet. It was shabby and had seen better days, but service and meals were still of a very high standard. The latter being formal affairs were overseen by the charming and well-travelled elderly Indian hostess, just as she had done for the previous fifty years when the British flocked to the coolness of the hill stations to escape the suffocating Indian summer. We rose early to view the sunrise over the snow-covered peak of Mt Everest, visited a tea plantation and the training school for Sherpa mountain guides. It was initiated and run by the Sherpa guide Tenzing Norgay, who had accompanied Sir Edmund Hillary at the time of conquering Everest in 1953 - announced the day of Queen Elizabeth's Coronation when I was sitting outside the Abbey. We declined an invitation to speak with him as time was pressing. We left India with lingering memories; extreme poverty, a kaleidoscope of colours, confusion everywhere, busy streets with cows and rickshaws, airline staff struggling with new computer systems, and the inadequacies of post offices and banks where staff recorded transactions in pencil in grubby exercise books. We savoured the aromas of tongue-tingling and sweet spices, and tolerated the unhygienic odours and unpleasant sights, which did not detract from our overall fascination for the country.

~o~

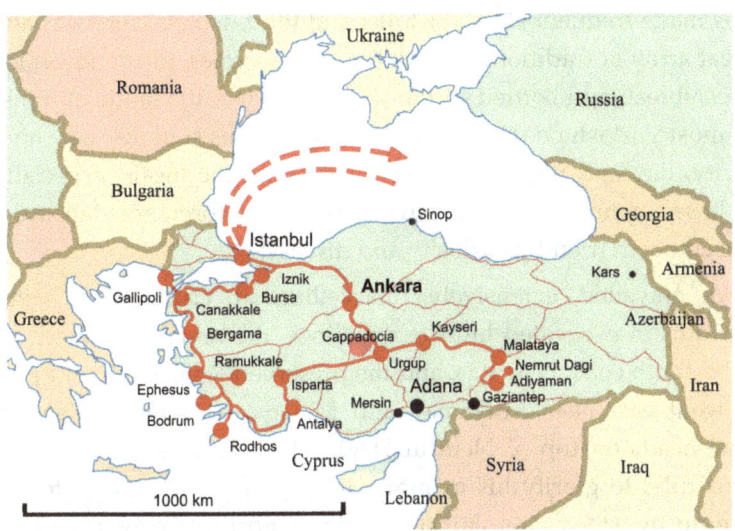

The Near East – our Turkey trip

Our five-week trip to Turkey in April 1991 was equally exciting, though not so colourful due to the sombre clothing worn by the Muslims. Again we immersed ourselves in the culture of this ancient civilisation, meeting the people and enjoying the local food at lokantas. We booked the first few nights in Istanbul and from then on stayed in Ottoman mansions and family-run B & Bs, relying on our bible and friend, Lonely Planet, or the ever-present touts who haunted the otogars (bus stations) pestering arriving passengers. As there was an airline strike and the trains were fully booked, we took an overnight bus from Istanbul to Ankara. It was the end of Ramadan when families gathered together as Christians do at Christmas. We enjoyed the experience so much, sitting high in the top of a double-decker bus where we were served drinks and chocolate biscuits on a pullout tray in front of us - rather like an aeroplane. We were blissfully unaware of the breakneck speed we were travelling at and the high incidence of bus accidents. We abandoned the idea of hiring a car in Ankara, and decided to continue our travels by the very cheap and efficient autobus - via a vast network stretching across the country. On long journeys buses made frequent stops for toilet and food, where there was always a great array of traditional and delicious casseroles, plus endless loaves of fresh bread and bottled spring water. This was the mode of transport that most Turkish people could afford, so the bus stations were hives of activity, day and night. Here we mixed with the locals, especially on the buses, when we were always the only foreigners aboard and aroused much friendly curiosity and discussion.

We travelled extensively, marvelling at Cappadocia with its labyrinths of excavated hillside dwellings, the remains of the lost city off the south coast near Kas, and the preserved Roman city of Ephesus. We went east near Adiyaman and Malatya, to view the enormous statue heads on top of Nemrut Dagi, which had been built by some minor ruler to glorify his memory. It was an unforgettable, terrifying drive up the steep mountainside, with a substitute driver, who could never pass a learner's test. He was in no fit state either after celebrating the end of Ramadan with illicit alcohol. Despite all we survived and after climbing the last stretch were awestruck by the view below, of surrounding mountains midst clouds and the huge statues before us - some broken and lying on the ground. I was dreading the drive down but it was quick and easy without incident. We were intrigued by the custom of serving chai, (apple tea was a great favourite) wherever one was in a bank queue, a pharmacy, or waiting in a dolbus queue.

We found the mountainous country very beautiful, especially as we saw it with red poppies in full bloom on the plains. At the entrance to each town, no matter how poor or small, it seemed there was a garden of flowering rose bushes between the lanes. One town in the mountains, Isparta, traded solely in rose products of every description. On entering the town we were blinded by pink on all sides. The stalls and shops were all decked out in a hectic pink and selling nothing but pink things. Perfumes, soaps, hair and skin products, jam, sweets, potpourri, essence, pictures, and crafts, the variety extended beyond the imagination and all rose-based and packaged in bright pink. The old ornate shoe-shining kits fascinated us; they were works of art in copper and proudly polished by their owners. At quays and terminals they were ever-present, and much in demand. At the quayside too, were fishmongers vying for business with their amazing displays. There also were flower sellers, and even with all the flowers we have in Australia, it struck me how bright the colours were - even more vivid than we see. We were surprised to see that the people used the mosques, not only for prayer, but as gathering places where women sat around gossiping and children played games. In Bursa, we saw one little boy in the pulpit chanting before a group of chattering laughing children.

When in Turkey I was continually reminded of the long history of Constantinople, and the country's glorious and turbulent past. Of course we visited all the wonders of past ages: the Blue Mosque, Topkapi Palace, the Spice and covered Grand Markets. From a ferry in the Bosphorus, we marvelled at the view of Istanbul with the spires of mosques dominating the city skyline at dusk. We took Turkish baths in Istanbul and Bursa in the west, and spent a few days on the island of Rhodos. We were very moved by our day trip to Gelliboli (Gallipoli), and touched by the Turks themselves and their sorrow over the tragedy.

~o~

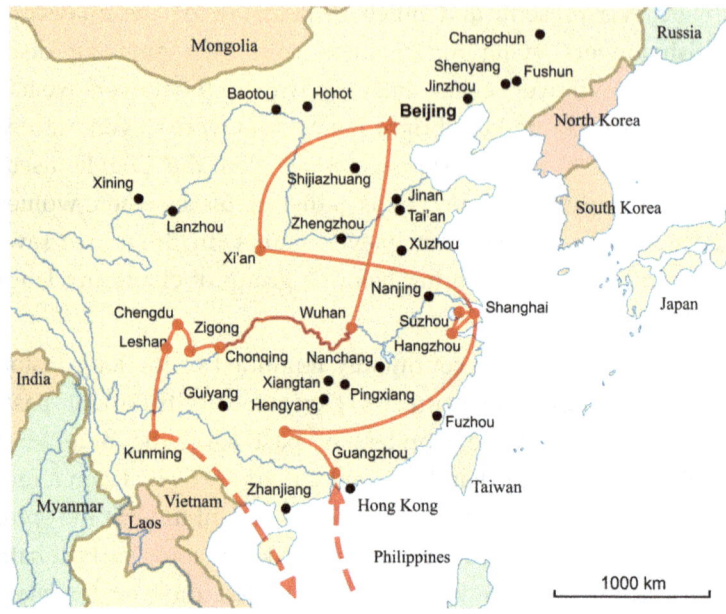

The Far East – our China trip

A few years later, we joined our friends Laurie and Jill Eadie on a guided tour to China with a group of twenty-two in total. It was extremely well organised, first class hotels with all tours and meals included, and very reasonably priced. The trip was only marred by our Australian guide, who was ignorant and insensitive. He was rude to two ladies, whom he threatened to send home, and to two undeserving local guides with threats of reporting them to their bosses (the government) and jeopardising their employment. All our Chinese guides were university educated, spoke excellent English, and were exceptionally intelligent with a great sense of humour. From Singapore we flew into Guangzhou, where we were met by Michael our Chinese guide for the first three of our four weeks in China. After viewing the wonderful museum and other sights, late in the day we boarded a China Airlines flight. As take-off was delayed, we were relieved when we landed safely in Guilin - considering the airline's poor accident record. We were lucky to make it to our cruise boat, as Guilin airport was under a sea of water when we left and no further flights came through for days.

Near Guilin we had a wondrous misty day on the river Li, where karst peaks rose high above the waterline. It was raining, which added to the magic, and I was moved to put pen to paper in the form of short poems. These poems continued, as I was inspired to write for the remainder of the trip.

Guilin – River Li

This floating world drifts and moves
Amidst the mists, where we are
But temporary visitors.

On to Shanghai: seventeen million people and as many bicycles and umbrellas in all colours of the rainbow. In the rain, people riding bicycles were shrouded in bright hooded capes. I was so impressed by the practicality and colourfulness of the capes that I bought some for our three children.

Shanghai – Who are they?

Who are they? These unknown figures
In their capes of many colours
Purple, blue, green and yellow
Silent, pedalling in each neat lane
To work, to home, we shall never know
Them, shrouded from the rain.

Here we walked along the infamous and once dangerous harbour front - The Bund. Now much changed, one of our party threw a cigarette butt into the harbour and was almost the subject of a citizen's arrest. We toured the protected, foreign embassy quarter, and walked in a beautiful Chinese garden with pavilions, lakes, bridges and ornamental trees and rocks; a pleasure that was repeated in other cities, though no two gardens were the same. It was in Shanghai that our Australian guide had an altercation with the two Margarets for lingering in a factory outlet shop, and unfairly blamed the Chinese guides when he lost his way in a street market.

In a disagreeable mood, our Australian guide eventually joined us for a traditional banquet in a restaurant frequented by all the locals. For the entire four weeks, we had Chinese banquets, such food as has never seen the West. Huge platters piled high with the most delicious variety of every imaginable vegetable and meat - the best food I have eaten anywhere in the world. From Shanghai, we caught a train bound for Hangzhou and although we had been warned about pick-pocketing in the crowded station, two of our group lost their wallets.

Hangzhou is a beautiful city with a man-made lake, in the centre of which there is an island. It was here we met a group of giggling small children, dressed in colourful clothing and on a school excursion.

Hangzhou – School Excursion Day

Little black heads patterned
In a kaleidoscope of colour
Happy round faces, laughing
In their colourful clothes
Bubbling, chattering
For it is school excursion day

We visited a tea plantation and sipped various teas, as is the Chinese custom - much as the appreciation and tasting of wine is in the western world. Some of us came away with their own special tea blend, costing a mere fifty US dollars for half a kilo! Outside our hotel we were accosted by chattering, pleading women eager to sell their local cultured pearl necklaces, and as the prices got progressively lower each time, we finally gave way to temptation before our departure.

Hangzhou – To Market

To market, to market
What shall we buy today?
Lawrie joins the Red Guard
Jill becomes a worker
Little M buys a ukelele
While Michael is the carrier
And Peter is the candy man.

To market, to market
What shall we buy today?
Silk scarves, jade or tea
Postcards, ties, cloisonné
Julie has an eye for pearls
Warren buys another strand
For his sweet lady fair.

To market, to market
What shall we buy today?
Quickly, quickly, time is short
As bags are getting very full
And Little M's in a quandary
What to do, with what she's bought
Michael's getting very fraught
'Ship off home!', is his retort.

Hangzhou – Stranger

Who is this stranger?
Like a stone breaks

A tranquil stream
Into a swirling pool
Of splintered colour.

Hangzhou – Farewell Songs by Huang

Sing to us, Huang
Your song of Edelweiss
Your songs of China
In your dulcet, lilting voice.

Mouth the words, oh Margaret
In such sweet silent tone
For Huang knows the words
He sings for us alone.

We went by bus to Suzhou, once called the Venice of The East due to the many beautiful bridges along the Grand Canal, which threads its way through the city. They once numbered more than four hundred, I believe. This man-made waterway was once a significant thoroughfare, extending from Peking to Nanking and used for the transportation of people, animals, produce, all goods, construction materials and so on, until the nineteenth century. Suzhou is noted for its gardens and one through which we walked consisted of three islands connected by delightful bridges. We viewed a very long and detailed antique scroll, which depicted the once busy canal complete with barges, and with descriptions of the villages along the entire route. Painted in the traditional Chinese vertical style, it was truly amazing. We were taken by barge along a section of the canal system and passed under a few of the last remaining bridges. All were in a state of decay as were the houses facing onto the canal; there was rubbish everywhere.

From Suzhou, we took a plane north-west to Xian and a true wonder of the world, the Terracotta Warriors that were accidentally uncovered by two farmers in a field in 1974. Further excavations revealed a vast army of life-size soldiers and horses in battle formation, made from clay and fired to terracotta in special kilns. No two soldiers or horses were alike. They were ordered by Qin Shi Huang, the first emperor, in 246 BC to protect him in his tomb.

Xian – Dumpling Banquet

Dumplings, dumplings
Anyone for dumplings?
Small, round, take your pick
Big and fat, thin or thick
Stuffed or not
No matter what
Sweet or sour
Gotta be quick!

Xian – Terracotta Warriors

Oh! Mighty noble warriors
Uncovered from the past
For two thousand years
You've served your Emperor well.

We flew next to Beijing, a city that impressed us with its lattice of wide freeways. Surprised by this general modernisation on one hand, the city was losing its Chinese character. I imagine now that in preparation for the Olympics, it is fast becoming like Los Angeles. Most impressive were the vast Tiananmen Square and the extensive Forbidden City. Armed soldiers were on duty everywhere and we saw them goose-stepping in formation when changing guard. We were given a comprehensive tour of the beautiful palace buildings, showing us both the luxury and the darker side of life in the time of the emperors. We were intrigued by the long queue of the faithful waiting to view Mao's tomb, and shuddered at the thought of the massacre of students protesting against the regime in 1989.

A magnificent solid marble boat was built for the last empress in the early twentieth century. Decorative rather than seaworthy, it was moored on sculpted dry canals providing an imaginary vista for her pleasure. We also saw the house where she imprisoned the child emperor and walked through the grounds of her palace.

Wonder-of-wonders is the Great Wall and even when some distance away, I was in awe of the wall with its watchtower forts stretching far over the hills ahead. It was a thrill to walk on the wall and to climb the steps where they were intact and safe.

Beijing – Great Wall

Great Wall, you beckon us
From afar, we have come
We stand before you,
In disbelief.
Can it be?
You too have travelled,
Long and far.

Ten of our group took a four-day cruise on the Yangtze River, from Wuhan to Chengdu. With accommodation for up to 140 on the boat and as many crew, our tiny group was the only one on board. We were thoroughly spoiled. We spent much time on deck including the early hours when going through the three gorges. We went ashore to visit villages en route and were saddened to learn of the millions, who would lose their homes and livelihoods after the damming of the river. There was karaoke and other entertainment every night, and at the end of the voyage, a magnificent Chinese banquet with courses presented in the shapes of swans, frogs, elephants and boats.

Yangtze River – On the 'China Glory'

Oh Captain Chang! Oh Mr Chang!
We are so very grateful for
Such generous hospitality
We have at our disposal
Your full complement of crew
No less than eight and eighty
To serve our every need
No matter what we choose to do
This Aussie group of ten

Oh Mr Hopson! Oh Mr Hopson!
Every morning we await your call
Oh Mr Hopson! Oh Mr Hopson!
We are forever at your beck and call
Each day, you delight us
By wanting to invite us
Tea, coffee, wine or banquet
Or some tantalising junket

Oh China Glory! Oh China Glory!
You have shared with us your history
We have viewed your wondrous gorges
From the decks of China Glory.
To have seen this ancient kingdom
We shall be ever grateful
And not forget your country
Returning home, China in our memory

Mini Gorges

What God created this masterpiece?
Winding through an ancient land
Sculptured by weather, flood and time
Sheer ochre cliffs fringed with green
Ribboned orange, black, golden dye,
Reaching to a heavenly sky
From turquoise water far below
Jewels of stone catch the eye
Beneath waters transparent, shallow

~o~

Other travels

[Ed. June was passionate about travelling - most of which was shared with Errol. She explored every nook and cranny of the cities she called home, toured most regions of the countries she lived in, and threw in cultured and exotic travel for the experience and to satisfy her curiosity. Together they often went back to see something they hadn't quite got to the first time, to relive memories, or visit dear friends. Errol is certain she would have written much more here had her physical capacities allowed it.]

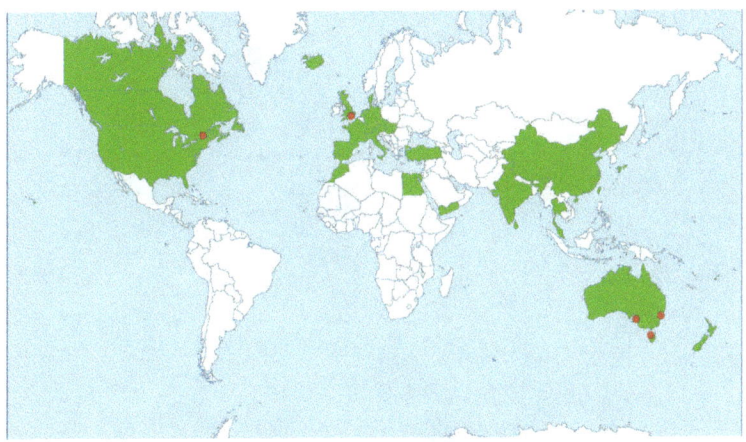

Residences and countries explored.

Following our trip to the Czech Republic, we returned the favour to our Czech hosts the following year. We have continued to meet regularly with our fellow travellers and established lasting friendships.

Other trips from Sydney were made to WA for three weeks with Fuff to view the wonderful wildflowers; to brother Guy's funeral (d. 5/9/1993, Burra); and to sister Peg's funeral (d. 24/2/1995).

~o~

My Silent Years

The Onset of MND

At the close of the twentieth century and approaching my seventy-fifth year, I entered the last phase and biggest challenge of my entire life. In December of 1999, Errol and I were visiting Jennifer in Hobart. She wanted me to join her in a singing workshop, but I detected a very slight hesitation in my speech. Barely perceptible Jennifer did notice it too. The following month it was apparent that something was wrong when my voice became quite husky. I could not sing and from then on, month-by-month, my voice became huskier and weaker, and I found myself hesitating in pronouncing words.

From February 2000 and well into 2001, I averaged two or three appointments a week with doctors of every known and unknown specialty, therapists of various sorts, and of course my GP. As well, I was constantly undergoing tests to determine the cause of my symptoms and treatments to ease the problem. I was first referred to an ear, nose and throat specialist, a neurologist and a gastroenterologist, who performed a gastroscopy. This went on for months, during which time I had barium swallows, EEG, ECG, X-rays and MRI scans of brain, throat, chest and lungs - all showing no abnormality for my age. However, my blood tests shared some indications with typical myasthenia gravis sufferers, thereby opening a line of investigation that was pursued fruitlessly for two years. In all I saw more than fifteen specialists, ranging from neurologist (five), the ENT, gastroenterologist, rheumatologist, immunologist, lung, goitre (did an arthroscopy) and others! As well, there were numerous speech therapists (more barium swallows), physiotherapists, a dietician, and an osteopathologist. The list was endless and was not to stop there. I felt that Errol and I had a new time-consuming and obsessive hobby, but it was nowhere near as pleasant.

The treatments for myasthenia ranged from Mestinon, Prednisone (cortisone) for more than a year, and other drugs to assist in putting the disease in remission – perhaps only for months or maybe for years. I had a Tensilon test in Concord Hospital, which partly discounted the myasthenia theory. As a last resort, I commenced five-day courses at Westmead Hospital of blood plasma exchange, where plasma is taken out, washed and returned to the body over a three-hour period. After three trials I showed no improvement, leading the head immunologist to the conclusion that I had Motor Neurone Disease (MND). Despite this my neurologist continued treating me for myasthenia gravis with higher doses of Prednisone, and as before, checking my hands and tongue for tremors - often early symptoms of MND. In January 2001 dissatisfied with my progress, Jennifer made an appointment with a Hobart neurologist, Bruce Taylor. He was very competent, examined all my records, thoroughly checked me out and did further testing in hospital the following day. He was in no doubt that I had motor neurone disease, and advised my Sydney neurologist of his findings and suggested I discontinue all drugs useless for treating MND.

My neurologist ignored this advice and asked whether Bruce Taylor was as old as himself, leading me to believe that he thought Dr Taylor might be inexperienced! Still on Prednisone with six weekly appointments, it was obvious that I was getting nowhere. The following June in desperation, I asked for a referral to Dr Pamphlett in the MND clinic at the Royal Prince Alfred Hospital. A month later, I had an appointment and after going through the usual history and testing, he too diagnosed MND. I returned for electrical tests on my nervous system before being referred on to Dominic Rowe, the MND specialist at the Royal North Shore Hospital (RNS), who finally confirmed my condition as a rare form of the disease.

Dominic is a very caring, knowledgeable, and handsome young neurologist, who agreed with the diagnosis. Incidentally, he knew Bruce Taylor and remarked that he was outstanding in his field, and had a practice in Melbourne as well as Hobart. As it happens, he was probably around forty or under, for Jennifer remembers him at university. Dr Rowe suggested I join his trials for saliva control, whereby he injected botox into the saliva glands. These were done fortnightly for some weeks and though successful to a point, they did not stop the saliva entirely. Months later, he came to our home to give another injection but as the effects are short-lived, I am now in need of more.

As with all specialists it takes time to get an appointment, so it was not until October 2001 when I first saw Dr Rowe and had a definite diagnosis. Until July of that year, I had not shown any of the weakness associated with MND. I was walking well and doing housework, even down on my hands and knees polishing the kitchen floor. In August, I did however slip on the stairs whilst carrying a tray downstairs, very cleverly spilling only water though shedding a bountiful supply of blood from a badly grazed leg. I was fit enough then to spend hours cleaning blood from the carpet. Fuff was staying with us and a district nurse was calling to dress a wound on her leg, so the nurse tended to my needs also. After high doses of Prednisone, my blood and skin were very thin with the result that the bad wound took months to heal. In the next few months though still walking, my legs showed signs of weakness and I became unsteady on my feet. Thereafter I used a walker to prevent further falls, and when going up and down stairs was sure to hold onto the rails.

In February of this year, 2002, I went into the RNS for a 'PEG' (Percutaneous Endoscopic Gastrostomy), which is used for taking food directly into the stomach. Cameron Bell inserted it under the supervision of Dominic Rowe and his competent, caring clinic staff. For the first eighteen months until July of last year, I continued with my other interests, selling my cards and attending my language classes, Japanese, French and Spanish – all up for about a year after I lost my voice completely. I did all my homework on the computer, took printouts to class where I was happy to listen, and wrote on paper when required to participate. My teachers Cella and Miyako, and fellow classmates were most sympathetic, enabling me to keep up my social contacts and interests. Miyako even drove me to class when I could no longer drive, due to yet another problem, a corneal graft and cataract removal, which I had done in December 2000. Errol took me to

Queensland for the graft operation and though successful, the recovery took twelve months and now the other eye has the same problems. With my reading ability affected, I had yet another handicap!

From early on, as well as my funny voice, my mouth muscles became very weak - particularly on the right side. This resulted in my jaw being thrown out, much like a stroke victim, and hence I continually bite my lips, tongue and inside of my cheeks. At a cost of $600, my dentist made a mouthguard for night use. It was highly successful until I feared choking - so discarded it. The continual flow of saliva has been the bane of my life and together with the biting, is almost worse than the loss of voice. The embarrassment of constant dribbling and stuffing a tissue in my mouth is still hard to bear, and although friends are so kind they have to try to not notice. When I see myself in the mirror, I can't believe what I see before me, an old, slumped, gaunt woman with mouth hanging open and staring lifeless eyes. Though my family contradict me, I feel I look years older than my aunts Jess and Kath when they died, aged one-hundred-and-one and ninety-seven respectively.

I have deteriorated so much in the last twelve months since not being able to walk, and there has been an associated loss of muscle in both my body and legs. During a spell in a respite hospital, I sat slouched in a chair for nine hours with nothing to do except gaze at the door, and was put to bed at seven. It was a debilitating and humiliating experience.

It is September 2002 and Ross has found a mini-disc recording from February of last year. He had just returned from Mexico and we, Errol, Ross and I, were discussing his purchases and the visit to Australia of Nicky and Leslie Minns. There was then a definite hesitation and change in my speaking pitch that is noticeable to those that know me well. To my knowledge, it is the only recording of me, and the first time I have heard my voice since I lost the ability to speak two years ago. While I was happy to hear my voice again, I felt very sad that I could no longer participate fully or make the odd passing comment as before. For some considerable time after my complete loss of speech, I communicated with pen and paper, and so was obliged to carry pads of recycled paper everywhere I went. I got through reams, particularly when answering questions for every new specialist I saw. Despite the fact that they had a detailed file of my history, they all wanted to hear it straight from the horse's mouth. I supplemented this by using a Lightwriter (a purpose-built notebook computer for displaying and speaking typed messages), in one-to-one conversations and on the telephone. For handling incoming calls, I pre-programmed some standard answers and conversational questions, and became very adept. Unfortunately, many people of my generation had trouble understanding the electronic voice, and were put off by the American accent. Next, I resorted to writing on a small whiteboard, and in the last few weeks as writing has become impossible, I point to a letter board spelling out words letter-by-letter. It is frustrating for both the reader, and me, and some are more patient than others. Most people expect a 'Yes' or 'No' answer to their questions, and yet phrase questions in such a way that a yes or no would be open to misinterpretation. Without further qualification, invariably, I am misunderstood. Others wildly guess, jump to conclusions, or worse still won't give me the letter board, which leads to confusion and frustration on both sides. I feel so helpless when I have an active mind and am treated like a nonentity - a vegetable. I wish I had Alzheimers and my GP agreed that it would be an easier cross to bear.

We have some wonderful, concerned friends visiting, who cheer me up, make me laugh and treat me quite normally. By contrast, some well-meaning people persist in standing close, shouting, talking slowly, or tell me who they are as one would to a senile or demented person. They may then go on to explain in great detail, something that I recollect or may know more about than they. I found it particularly upsetting, when one sister in the respite hospital refused to let me write, nor would she read any message because she did not have time. Yet she herself talked non-stop about how busy they were, which was true, and other less important things; all the while wasting my opportunity to communicate directly. She went to great length to explain how gravity works, and after warning me of the dangers of aspiration (something I was well aware of), she promptly poured a drink straight down my throat while I was lying down. Of course, it went down the wrong way! I was treated as dim-witted though she knew I was not, and she always knew more about my condition and needs than I did – and worse, she was invariably wrong. I can well understand now why some patients lose control and turn violent, as at times I came very close to screaming the place down and would have struck that woman had I been able. Had I done so, I imagine I would have been put in a straitjacket and regarded as unmanageable.

It really is so humiliating to be treated in such a way and then so undignified to lose control. At other times and despite being in continuing pain, I do not even feel sorry for myself. All I want is an understanding of this dreadful disease, but mainly to be happy and not be a nuisance to others in my final days. My loving family give support in every possible way, and all nurses and carers, who come to our home, are truly caring, patient and kind. As mentioned before, friends from far and wide visit bearing flowers, food, good cheer and other assistance, which help Errol and me to carry on. The PEG feeding tube was inserted in my stomach last February, as a precaution should I have more difficulty in swallowing, and while my heart and lungs were strong enough to withstand the operation. Up to the present time 22nd October 2002, and almost three years since I first noticed changes in my speech, it is only used for water and medications. I am still able to eat by mouth and so share tasty foods after modifying their consistency, by blending or adding yoghurt, cottage cheese or sauces.

Even my loving family do not always understand all of my problems. When I make a noise it is not necessarily because I am seeking attention but could be one of many things; I may have bitten my lip, tongue or cheek and am in pain that is now more intense, or be trying to pick up something that is out of reach or that I have dropped. For two years, the only sounds I have been able to make are grunts or a sort of cry, which can turn into an uncontrollable shriek or a cackle when I laugh. It is very hurtful to be mimicked or to be told not to grunt. Worse still, I have been accused of wailing and whingeing. One physiotherapist even told me not to look so severe and to smile at my husband; unfortunately, I cannot change the former, nor can I do the latter.

I notice that as each day passes, I lose more muscle strength and movement in my back, legs and especially arms, hands and fingers. This has lead in the last few days (20th November 2002), to much difficulty in pointing to letters, picking up even tissues, reaching, pressing and typing. As well for one and a half years, I have been unable to blow my nose, suck through a straw, spit out, all of which the majority of nurses cannot comprehend. For some time, it has been very hard to reach to scratch myself anywhere on my body, and my skin is so sensitive that I seem to itch all over. My reach too is now limited to my nose. The average person has no idea just how often they scratch themselves, or how frustrating it is to leave a persistent and nagging itch.

Now it is a struggle to keep going, as I am losing the ability to type and people do not have time or patience to read the letter board. I have battled and persevered for so long to hang on, in order to express myself, enjoy the taste of food, the company of friends, and the better news and entertainment programs available via the electronic media. Little did I know back in January 2000 how serious my problem would prove to be, or the effect it would have upon me and my family, I still don't know for how many years to come. Despite all, in the last eighteen months while ill I realised two substantial goals, which I had had in mind for many years.

Against all odds - entering the Wynne

In March of 2001, within ten days, I completed two large sculptural landscape paintings for the Wynne Prize, I got started with much encouragement from Trevor, who surprised me with the registration forms and then helped me choose the subject matter. He then flew from Melbourne for a weekend to make the complicated three-dimensional frames. While I continued working from morning till night, Jennifer arrived for a week from Hobart to take over all cooking and household duties, plus setting up and cleaning all my equipment each day. Of course, Errol ably assisted the enthusiastic team. Being multimedia paintings, I used plaster of Paris to build up the layers of the topography, hessian for texture and coloured inks for my abstract depictions of the Escarpment at Kakadu Gorge, and the Bungle Bungles in WA.

Eighty-six thousand words

My other notable achievement is that in February of this year 2002, I started writing my memoirs. Now almost a year later, I have more than 86,000 words behind me and am basically finished. I hope they serve to inform my children of my life and of the times in which I grew up. Despite writing only a few lines each day, it has been enormously satisfying and filled in my solitary days. At the present time, I am attempting to fill in gaps and assist with obvious corrections and the editing.

Most importantly, since they learnt of my illness, I have been genuinely touched by the sincere and loving kindness shown by many people, often from sources least expected.

Haikus from nature

[Ed. Unable to sleep due to frequent cramping, June distracted herself by composing haikus. First opportunity in the morning, she would relay them to family or carers. She focussed on letters on a transparent sight-board while the reader followed her eye movements. June derived much inspiration from nature and especially the beautiful surrounds of her home.]

Dead tree trunks once grey
rising sun turn to silver
briefly come alive

Outside my window
bamboo arch welcomes each day
twenty years and more

My Silent Years

Camellias bloom
shades of pink, red, white bring
cheer / life passes me by

Trickling stream gurgles
brings music to dreams by night
dreams of days long past

Fern fronds stirred by
gentle breeze, welcome the day
wave me good morning

Parched dry earth wilts
rain comes, elephants ears
proudly lift their heads

Dry creek comes to life
sudden rain rushing water
is joy to my ears

Rain pitter-patters
happy birds chirp and chatter
spring is here again

Sunlight filters through
trees form patterns and free
imagination

Little kumquat balls
small orange suns midst green
light up dull winter days

White ghost gum stands tall
overlooks his native cousins
king of the forest

Bamboo leaves float like
butterflies flutter and fall
to restore the earth

Noisy birds alert
gathering storm clouds burst forth
quench the thirsty earth

Temperatures rise
drought scorched earth bushfires
rage destruction sadness

Brown leaves on the ground
long past their autumn glory
crackle under foot

Origami cranes
in kaleidoscope colours
whirl before my eyes

A Quality Life

Sit contemplating
thoughts gather in my mind
no way to express

Stirred by rising wind
giant tree ferns wave their fronds
is it an omen

Throughout the long night
stifling pain, compose haiku
waiting for the dawn

~o~

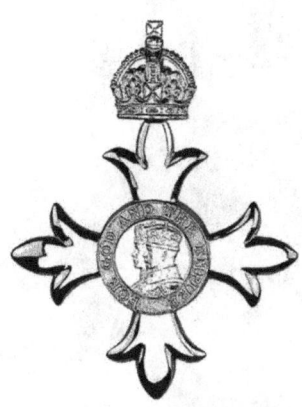

The Old Bugger's Eighty

[Ed. Simon Gentry presented Errol with an OBE (was actually a Golden Rough). The following transcript was read for June at the party, Finlay Rd, Warrawee. Sunday, 1st September 2002.]

'Since the start of our courtship fifty-one years ago in the small town of Burra, when you courted me with an inundation of flowers, (not to mention the ten shilling note), and we corresponded by snail mail for eighteen months until I joined you in Montreal, where we were married after a long separation, (incidentally, the day following my arrival) … you have been my staff and rod through the years, never more true than now.

Despite the ups and downs over forty-nine years, we HAVE survived, and above all are blessed with the most precious gift of all, three wonderful caring and loving children, who could not have been conceived without JUST a little input from you.

You have continued to present me with flowers, and above all, you have carried the recent burden of caring for me with devotion, for which I thank you. 'HAPPY BIRTHDAY MY DEAREST ERROL - MAY YOU HAVE MANY HAPPY HEALTHY YEARS AHEAD'

~o~

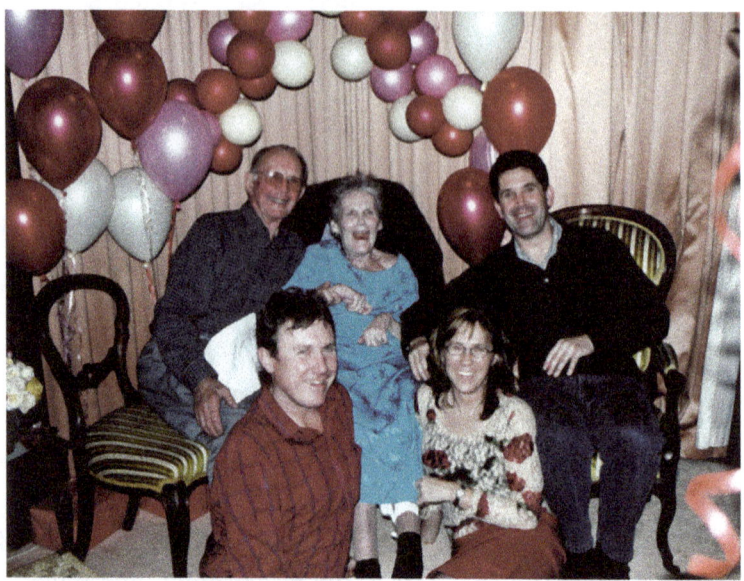

My 77th birthday party

[Ed. Sunday 15th June 2003. Friends and family gathered at Finlay Rd for June's last birthday party. Expertly made up (and PEG bag hidden by the drapes), she received her guests downstairs. June had her own surprise. She had composed a personal haiku for everyone, together with some less charitable after respite care at Wahroonga, and a treasured escape to the park opposite with me - Trevor. This is how she is remembered: proud, defiant and a great deal of fun to be around.]

Balloons flowers friends
family, queen on her throne
Happy Birthday June!

Ross like a mother
tends my every need
with patience and care

Cradled like a babe
in his arms Ross lifts me high
into a dream world

My Silent Years

Trevor eldest child
ever committed to our
family welfare

Devoted Errol
love, care with dedication
eases my burden

Darling Jenny Wren
thoughtful presents letters cards
visits from Hobart

Ups downs funny sides
assumptions misconceptions
being a veggie

Good doggie quiet sit up
shush paws down
doggie get your bone

Trailing violets
hang in window gift from Kate
my Gemini twin

Pat Buckle actress
comedienne anecdotes
wit make me chuckle

Bearing flowers, gifts
stories, massage, Margaret my
sister of charity

Lady Evelyn
perfumed roses, dinners, bridge
with Sir Eric

Jock Gwen long-time friends
happy times, parties, tennis
debating with Jock

Paradise is in
Dorrigo Cairnes* gourmet chefs
a 5-star resort   *(Doris, Peter)

Czech Republic met
jolly Gentrys shared bathroom
gin dumplings galore

Pain pain go away
do not torment me so, come
nightfall sleep and peace

Fuffy big sister
my angel watching over
me throughout my life

A Quality Life

Family, friends, carers
nurses. I count my lucky stars
surrounded by love

Two chooks heads chopped off
unnamed ladies handling hoist
a comical sight

In my chariot
through the park birds calling
a twilight escape

Bushwalking round and
around the lords of the forest
looking at the moon

Danusha Polish
beauty flamboyant divine
diva has run away

Polly and Kate
favourite team much giggling
a good start to my day

On my bedroom wall
three little lambs glow at night
send me off to sleep

No words to express
my thoughts, feelings and my
dreams / can't cry silently

Joybells and Ken
Rob, Peter, Bronny close-knit
happy family

Lovely Leanne
compassionate, like Erene
a perfectionist

Inside my window
thoughtful Erene creates a
garden of beauty

Good-natured Tracey
always cheerful patient Renee
make life worth living

~o~

Index

Associations: Baby Health Centre, 191; Baldwin Street International Tennis Club, 222, 236; Masonic Lodge, 64; Monkland Tennis Club, 133; Red Cross, 191; Royal Automobile Association, 10; South Australian Jockey Club, 25; Victoria League, 95, 108, 191; Youth Hostel, 96; YWCA, 59, 140

Education: Burra School 150th Anniversary, 30; Certificate; Art, 203; Ceramics, 202; French Proficiency, 140; Intermediate, 39; Leaving, 39; Tasmanian Teachers Certificate, 210, 211; Hellyer College, 217; **Language Study;** French, 39, 79, 140, 227, 228, 257; German, 39, 227; Japanese, 154, 226, 227, 228, 257; Latin, 39; Spanish, 228, 257; Launceston College, 209; Miss Mann's Business College, 25; Museum of Montreal, 137; Parklands High School, 202; Scotch College, 70; St Martin in the Fields, 107; St Mary's Sunday School, 29; St Peter's College, 36, 38; Tertiary; Macquarie University, 226; Tasmanian College of Advanced Education, 208; University of the Third Age, 228; The Wilderness School, 29; Woodlands CEGGS, 33, 38, 41, 53, 62, 107

Events: 21st Birthday Party, 54; Archibald, Wynne & Sulman Prizes, 205, 261; Burra Show, 7, 53; China Olympics, 249; Communion, 52; Courtship, 46, 57, 59, 61, 63, 65, 66; Engaged - not quite, 58; First boyfriend, 53; First real kiss, 53; Eastman Kodak Errol colour blind, 129; Edinburgh Tattoo, 99; Elegance Dinners, 223; Farnborough Air Show, 110; King Neptune Dunking, 76; Melbourne Cup, 182; Michael Crawford,Billy, 149; **Motor Neurone Disease**; Diagnosis, 257; MND Clinic, 256; Onset, 255; PEG, 257; Tests, 256; Mt Everest Conquered, 116; Octopussy, 239; Olympics, 130; Portia Geach Prize, 205; Queen Elizabeth Coronation, 109, 116, 240; Queen Elizabeth Garden Party, 120; Royal Adelaide Show, 57; Royal Sydney Easter Show, 222; Showcase, 223; Swan Lake with Rudolph Nureyev, 205; Tatler Pages, 109, 110; The Beaufort Hunt, 109; The Proms at Albert Hall, 106; Victory Day, 49; **War;** The Rockets, 43; **Wedding**, 125, 126; Gifts, 118, 119; Honeymoon, 127, 131; Outfits, 119

Family: Burdon, Errol Rex, 26, 46, 59, 61, 63, 64, 65, 70, 71, 73, 77, 79, 97, 103, 108, 115, 118, 119, 122, 125, 126, 127, 128, 129, 132, 133, 134, 135, 137, 139, 141, 145, 147, 148, 149, 150, 152, 154, 155, 156, 157, 158, 160, 161, 162, 175, 176, 177, 178, 179, 180, 181, 183, 188, 189, 193, 195, 196, 197, 200, 201, 202, 204, 210, 211, 212, 214, 215, 216, 219, 220, 221, 222, 224, 226, 227, 229, 230, 231, 232, 235, 255, 257, 258, 260, 262, 265, 267; **Burdon, Jennifer Margaret**, 70, 143, 147, 148, 151, 156, 178, 184, 186, 189, 190, 198, 199, 201, 202, 204, 207, 208, 212, 216, 217, 219, 221, 230, 231, 232, 233, 255, 256, 261, 267; **Burdon, Petrina June**, 179, 193, 195, 196, 202; **Burdon, Ross Andrew**, 27, 53, 55, 114, 126, 143, 147, 151, 159, 160, 161, 162, 175, 176, 177, 181, 184, 197, 198, 199, 202, 204, 207, 208, 209, 212, 216, 220, 222, 230, 231, 232, 235, 258, 266; **Burdon, Trevor Leslie**, 78, 126, 143, 145, 147, 151, 158, 159, 160, 175, 176, 193, 197, 198, 199, 201, 204, 205, 206, 207, 208, 209, 212, 217, 220, 221, 229, 232, 238, 261, 267

Holidays: Australia-Northern Territory; Alice Springs, 231; Darwin, 231; Kakadu, 231; Uluru, 231; **Australia-South Australia**; Oulnina Park, 231; Wilpena Pound, 231;

269

A QUALITY LIFE

Australia-Tasmania; Flinders Island, 232; **Australia-Victoria**; Malacoota, 230; **Australia-Western Australia**, 253; **Austria**, 236, 237; **Bali**; Kuta Beach, 231; Sanur, 231; Ubud, 231; **Canada**; Halifax, 154; Montreal, 236; Niagara Falls, 128; Nova Scotia, 154; Ontario, 129, 150; Prince Edward Island, 154; Toronto, 129, 148; **China**, 237, 244, 251; Beijing, 249, 250; Chengdu, 250; Great Wall, 78; Guilin, 244, 245; Hangzhou, 246, 247, 248; Nanking, 248; Peking, 248; River Li, 245; Shanghai, 245, 246; Suzhou, 248; Terracotta Warriors, 78, 248, 249; Tiananmen Square, 249; Wuhan, 250; Xian, 78, 248, 249; Yangtze River, 250, 251; **Czech Republic**, 237, 253, 267; **Egypt**, 155, 235; Abu Simbel, 235; Aswan Dam, 235; Cheops Grand Pyramid, 235; Luxor, 235; Pyramids, 239; Saqqara, 235; **Europe**, 96, 235, 236, 237; **France**, 78, 236; Avignon, 80; Marseilles, 79; Notre Dame, 78; Paris, 78, 236; **Greece**; Parthenon, 239; **Holland**, 235, 236; Amsterdam, 235; **Hong Kong**, 215; **Hungary**, 237; **India**, 155, 200, 237, 238, 239, 240; Ajunta, 239; Dahl Lake, 239; Darjeeling, 239; Hotel Windermere, 239; Jaipur, 239; Kashmir, 239; Lake Palace, 238; Mt Everest, 240; Rajasthan, 239; Rumbagh Palace, 239; Sherpa School, 240; Srinigar, 239; Taj Mahal, 239; Varanasi, 239; **Italy**, 236; **Japan**, 155, 215, 226, 237; Hakone, 216; Hokkaido, 226; Honshu, 227; Kyoto, 215; Sapporo, 226; Tokyo, 215; **Morocco**; Tangiers, 149; **New Zealand**, 216, 231; **North America**, 235; **Portugal**, 78; **Slovakia**, 237; **Spain**, 78, 228; Granada, 149; Malaga, 149; Ronda, 149; **Switzerland**, 236; **Taiwan**, 215; **Thailand**, 215; **Turkey**, 78, 131, 138, 237, 241, 243; Adiyaman, 138, 242; Ankara, 241; Bosphorus, 243; Bursa, 243; Ephesus, 242; Gallipoli, 243; Istanbul, 241, 243; Kas, 242; Malatya, 138, 242; Rhodos, 243; Topkapi, 243; **United Kingdom**; Exeter, 236; Firth of Forth, 99; Nottingham, 115; Nottingham Castle, 115; Perth, 99; Sherwood Forest, 115; **USA**; Appalachian Mountains, 130; Boston, 134; Detroit, 236; Eden Roc Hotel, 153; Everglades, 153; Florida, 153; Fontainbleu Hotel, 153; Guggenheim Museum, 143; Hampshire, 154; Hawaii, 235, 236; Lake Placid, 130; Las Vegas, 236; Maine, 142; Manhattan Island, 142; Miami Beach, 153; Rochester, 129; Rochester Center, 142; Rockport, 153; San Diego, 147, 236; Statue of Liberty, 143; Tiffanys, 143; United Nations, 142; Vermont, 130, 144, 148, 149; Washington, 138

Hospitals: Adelaide Children's hospital, 49; Burnie General Hospital, 189; Concord Hospital, 256; Hornsby Hospital, 227; Ku-ring-gai Hospital, 228; North-West General Hospital, 212; Perth Hospital, 195; Queen Victoria Hospital, 158; Royal Adelaide Hospital, 56, 57; Royal North Shore Hospital, 256, 257; Royal Prince Alfred Hospital, 256; Westmead Hospital, 256

People: Australia-New South Wales; Batache-Watt, Dr Emy, 228; Boyd, Gordon & Jillian, 223; Buckle, Patty & Red, 223, 267; Buddle, Jill, 226; Cairnes, Doris & Peter, 230, 267; Cordner, John & Gwen, 71, 217, 223, 236; Eadie, Jill, 226, 244; Humiko, 154; Jones, Joy & Ken, 268; Lewis, Mary & Keith, 222, 224; MacPherson, Anne & Jim, 223; Matsunaga, Kazuko, 226; Minton, Ken, 97; Miyako, 257; Moore, Red, 223; Pamphlett, Dr, 256; Phillips, Evelyn & Eric, 236, 267; Roden, June & Warwick, 229; Rowe, Dr, 67; Rowe, Dr Domenic, 256, 257; Rowe, Dr Dominic, 256, 257; Seiko, 226; **Australia-South Australia**; Avery, Uncle Lou, 215; Blesing, Rae, 67, 68, 69; Bowen, Audrey, 40, 51, 52, 53, 59; Bowen, Audrey 'Bunny', 144; Breeze, Bob, 15; Bryant, 1, 3, 27, 29, 47, 53, 112, 134, 149, 188, 190, 230; Bryant, Arthur Murray & Ernest Firth, 10, 21, 22; Bryant, Aunt Jess, 22, 26, 67, 93, 95, 96, 97, 105, 109, 110,

INDEX

111, 112, 116, 118, 119, 121, 122, 126; Bryant, Aunt Kath, 1, 3, 10, 21, 22, 23, 24, 25, 26, 33, 34, 35, 42, 57, 59, 60, 67, 70, 72, 97, 111, 113, 126, 152, 161, 178, 215, 231, 234, 235; Bryant, Aunt Nora, 15, 26, 42, 64; Bryant, 'Grandfather' George Benjamin, 3, 21, 23, 24, 25, 26, 29, 33, 35, 37, 47, 53, 55, 111, 112, 113; Bryant, 'Mum' Doris Mary, 1, 3, 4, 6, 9, 12, 13, 14, 15, 17, 18, 21, 23, 26, 27, 29, 30, 37, 49, 54, 57, 60, 61, 62, 66, 67, 68, 69, 70, 110, 178, 214, 215, 230; Bryant, Uncle Harry George, 22, 27; Burdon, Ivor, 61, 63, 65, 133, 141, 231; Burdon, Marlis & Peter, 231; Christie, Don, 53, 59, 67; Clark, Guy, 49; Clarke, Reg, 53; Culpin, June, 30, 54; Danslow, Paul, 45, 57; Davey, Clem, 4, 215; Davies, Diana & Joan, 40, 42; Dollman, 3, 9, 19, 27, 215, 230; Dollman, 'Dad' Guy Herbert, 1, 3, 4, 6, 7, 9, 10, 11, 12, 13, 14, 18, 20, 21, 24, 31, 33, 42, 43, 46, 49, 55, 56, 61, 62, 66, 68, 69, 70, 178, 214, 215, 230, 231; Dollman, Frances Jean 'Fuff', 1, 3, 6, 9, 10, 12, 13, 14, 15, 17, 20, 25, 26, 29, 31, 41, 45, 48, 49, 51, 53, 61, 68, 70, 112, 144, 178, 215, 216, 231, 253, 257; Dollman, 'Grandad' Ernest Guy, 4; Dollman, 'Grandma' Jane, 3, 4; Dollman, Guy Bryant, 7, 9, 14, 21, 26, 49, 70, 253; Dollman, Helen Valerie, 1, 9, 19, 29, 31, 40, 42, 43, 48, 49, 53, 67, 70, 194, 215; Dollman, Helen Valerie 'Tubby', 54; Dollman, Ruth Margaret 'Peg', 1, 4, 6, 12, 20, 25, 26, 29, 41, 43, 48, 52, 53, 54, 60, 70, 153, 215, 231, 253; Donaldson, Captain John, 96, 97, 105, 110, 112, 113, 118, 119, 121, 122; Donaldson, Catherine Frances, 9; Dow, Diana, 5, 6, 20; Dow, Diana & Graham, 4, 5, 9, 20, 31, 36; Dow, Myrtle, 20, 55; Dow, Reg, 36; Eason, Headmaster, 39, 107; Elsie, Housekeeper, 24, 111, 112, 113; Fraser, Don, 216; Fraser, Maxine 'Frizzy', 36; Glennister, Doris & Jack, 4, 9; Glennister, Mary Elizabeth, 9; Glennister, Ruth Grace, 9; Gurney, Ron, 57; Hastings, Don, 73; Hubert Opperman, 19; James, Jimmy, 5; Lehman, Ted, 43, 56, 65; Longford, Mervyn, 63; Mac, Chauffeur, 25; Marchants, 18; Marshall, Alan, 35; Matthews Store, 19; McHenry, Jeanette & Peter, 71; Miller, Cathy, 112; Miller, John, 111, 113; Miller, Uncle John, 26, 96, 122; Millington, Headmistress, 35; Miss Pearce, 6, 29, 30; Morgans, 20; Murdoch, Keith, 19; Neale, Jeff, 10; Nicholson, Bruce, 45; Oliver, Rev Canon, 126; Pearce, Norman, 18, 55; Redding, Major Donald 'Pop', 4, 5, 215; Richardson, Dulcie, 42; Rosman, Comedian Mr, 43; Sara & Dunstan, 29; Senior, Graham, 20; Sparrow, Nadine 'Spoggy', 39; Steele, Dr David, 1; Stevenson, Peg & Tom, 49; Storey, Frank, 15, 59; Terry, Jim, 67; Thomas, Jeanette, 71; Tye, Bob, 45; Walker, Alan, 61; White, Teacher Mrs, 32; Wincey, Cynthia, 1, 26, 236; Wincey, Deidre, 196; Wincey, Uncle Bill, 26; Winkie, 27; Wylie, Betty, 93, 109; **Australia-Tasmania**; Adams, Brian & Marlene, 185, 219; Atkins, Noel, 213; Cuatt, Lisa, 208; Duffield, Phyl & Bill, 216; Faulkner, Rosy, 213, 214; Fry, Win & Bill, 219; Gandy, Pam & John, 193; Gill, Andrew, 159, 192; Gill, Peggy & David, 190, 203, 212; Greenhill, Carol & Lance, 201; Harris, Lloyd, 184, 186; Haward, Phyllis & Dr Geoff, 208, 212; Haworth, Betty & Peter, 149; Hayes, Margaret & Warren, 78; Hiller, Kit, 205; Inglis, George, 215; Ingram, Dr Tom, 189, 193; Lauder, Ailee & Roy, 212; Lazenby, Nigel, 205; Leonard, Trevor, 207; Makin, Geoff, 202; Minns, Margaret & Derek, 78, 181, 187, 188, 189, 192, 194, 195, 212, 232, 258; Mitchell, Val & Bob, 213, 214; Neville, Joan & Royce, 159, 212; Nicholls, Frances & Nick, 182, 183, 191, 193; Nicholls, Margaret, 186; Proverbs, Kim & Roxanne, 204; Rainbird, Steve, 205, 213; Robinson, Shirley, 206; Rollins, Paul, 205; Rosewall, Ken, 187; Savage, Doff 'Dorothy', 70; Simpson, Leslie, 204; Simpson, Rita, 212; Spooky, 202; Stalker, Miss

A QUALITY LIFE

Winsome, 204; Sugars, Dr Keith, 216; Taylor, Dr Bruce, 256; Thorne, Headmaster Alan, 199; Turner, Alan, 203, 206; Turner, Rhoda, 210; Vynalek, Milan, 190; Wood, Jenny, 204; **Canada**; Bennett, Stella & Tony, 134, 162; Bentley, Norm & Midge, 143, 153, 236; Bentley, Tich, 143; Chamberlain, Dr Richard, 158; Ferrier, Wendy & Malcolm, 133, 134, 147, 236; Fotheringham, Ann & Walter, 152, 175, 176; Glencross, Jean & Eric, 149, 152; Goldberg, Eric, 140; Gray, Wendy & Ron, 143; Gregor, Yolan, 134, 157, 236; Halsey, Gwen & James, 145, 236; Harvey, Marie & Ed, 118, 150; Hewson, Doreen & Lorne, 150, 176; Knight, Claire & George, 134, 157; Laurie, Dymphna & John, 152, 244; Lester, Chairman, 146; Lismer, Dr Arthur, 137; McAsey, Inez & Ed, 125, 145; McLeod, Betty & Selby, 125, 139; Meagher, Mrs, 125, 162; Murphy, Ethel & Bryant, 134, 149, 204; Oliver, Rev Canon, 126; Oxorn, Dr Harry, 155, 156, 157, 158, 179; Parker, Johnnie, 149, 151; Perry, Dot & George, 133; Scholes, Bunny & John, 129, 148, 150, 152; Shannon, Geoff, 141, 144; Sheidow, Ann, 152; Spock, Dr, 158; Vicars, Gisele & Jack, 152; Ward, Miss, 18; Winnicki, Gwen, 144; Younghusband, Earl, 126; **United Kingdom**; Archdeacon, Margaret & Tony, 236; Begg, Dr, 32, 120; Delaney, Diana, 101, 113; Donaldson, Captain John, 96; Doyle, Arthur Conan, 94; Duke of Beaufort, 109; King George VI, 117; Lady Moyra Hamilton, 109; Norfolk Broads, 112; Prince Philip, 120; Prince Philip, Duke of Edinburgh, 120; Queen Elizabeth, 116; Queen Mother, 93, 100, 108, 117; Robin Hood, 115; Royal Family, 99, 116; Shakespeare, 97; Sherlock Holmes, 94; Wrixon-Becher, 108, 109, 110; Wylie, Betty & Hugh, 93; **USA**; Robert Louis Stevenson, 130

Places: Arabian Peninsula, 76; **Atlantic Ocean**, 80, 123; **Australia-New South Wales**, 9, 70, 230; Anthony Horderns, 178; Blue Mountains, 57, 229; Broken Hill, 9, 56, 59, 62, 63, 71, 93, 125, 230; Coonabarabran, 231; Dorrigo, 230, 267; Finlay Road, 220, 222, 226; Kings Cross, 60; Northbridge, 220; Pyrmont, 60; Southern Highlands, 229; St Ives, 228; Sydney, 9, 37, 42, 57, 59, 67, 70, 71, 97, 99, 107, 114, 123, 141, 145, 148, 176, 177, 178, 183, 202, 206, 209, 210, 212, 213, 215, 217, 219, 220, 221, 226, 227, 229, 230, 235, 256; Warrawee, 222; Wilcannia, 4, 9, 55, 230, 231; **Australia-Northern Territory**; Darwin, 42; Kakadu, 262; **Australia-Queensland**, 144; **Australia-South Australia**, 1, 9, 19, 25, 44, 47, 50, 55, 72, 95, 120, 141, 214; Adelaide, 1, 4, 9, 17, 19, 20, 21, 23, 24, 29, 32, 33, 34, 39, 43, 45, 47, 48, 49, 51, 54, 56, 57, 58, 60, 63, 64, 65, 67, 69, 70, 71, 72, 152, 177, 178, 180, 200, 215, 230, 231; Booborowie, 51, 61; Broadway Hotel, 47; Broadway, Glenelg, 23, 33, 42, 113; Burra, 1, 4, 5, 6, 7, 9, 12, 17, 26, 27, 29, 31, 33, 36, 39, 42, 45, 51, 52, 53, 54, 59, 61, 62, 63, 64, 65, 66, 107, 117, 120, 178, 215, 231, 265; Clare, 51, 63, 64; Eyre Peninsula, 26; Hanson, 51; Kooringa, 12, 14, 51, 59, 63; Orroroo, 231; Peterborough, 45; Port Adelaide, 26, 178; Port Lincoln, 26, 27; Port Pirie, 63, 125, 133; Port Wakefield, 12; Queen Street, 14, 59; Redruth, 12; River Murray, 27, 57; Saddleworth, 54; Semaphore Beach, 25, 26, 48, 51; St Mary's Church, 11, 17; Thames Street, 7, 12; Ware Street, 12, 18, 20; Waterfall Gully, 22; **Australia-Tasmania**, 70, 154, 179, 180, 185, 195, 207, 209, 211, 212, 214, 215, 217, 220, 226, 232; Australian Pulp and Paper Mill, 189, 201; Bass Strait, 180, 184, 232; Boat Harbour, 192, 193; Burnie, 181, 182, 183, 184, 189, 192, 195, 197, 199, 201, 202, 203, 204, 206, 210, 212, 213, 214, 215, 217, 219, 220; Derwent River, 141, 232; Devonport, 181, 204, 212; Hobart, 70, 141, 183, 195, 203, 206, 208, 209, 211, 212,

272

INDEX

213, 214, 215, 220, 221, 222, 232, 255, 256, 262, 267; Lactos Cheese, 190; Launceston, 62, 194, 196, 204, 206, 207, 208, 210, 212, 232, 233; Menai Hotel, 181, 186; Mt Wellington, 141; Penguin, 196; Salamanca Place, 214; Savage River Mines, 213; Seaview Avenue, 184, 212; Sulphur Creek, 201; Ulverstone, 182, 201; Wynyard, 192; **Australia-Victoria**; Melbourne, 45, 49, 51, 62, 63, 153, 177, 178, 194, 197, 201, 210, 261; **Australia-Western Australia**, 262; Bungle Bungles, 262; Kalgoorlie, 195; Perth, 72, 213; Tudor Court, 72; **Canada**, 41, 46, 47, 61, 65, 69, 70, 71, 72, 109, 115, 117, 118, 121, 123, 125, 127, 129, 131, 137, 138, 139, 146, 147, 148, 149, 152, 154, 178, 209, 234; Algonquin, 127, 128; Beaconsfield, 161; Cote St Luc, 140, 146; Jacques Cartier Bridge, 132, 148; Labrador Peninsula, 123; Lachine, 149; Lake Champlain, 131, 139, 142; Lake Louise, 127; Lake Memphremagog, 153; Lake Paquin, 151; Lakes District, 112, 236; Lakeshore, 125, 141, 146, 161; Laurentian Mountains, 139, 144; Le Château Frontenac, 127; Magill University, 132; Monkland Avenue, 145, 146, 155; Montreal, 118, 119, 122, 123, 125, 132, 134, 136, 140, 141, 142, 143, 144, 146, 149, 150, 151, 152, 162, 176, 177, 179, 189, 227, 265; Mount Royal, 123, 140; Museum of Montreal, 132; Newfoundland, 123, 144; Notre Dame, 145; Notre Dame de Grace, 125; Ontario, 151, 162; Ottawa, 126, 127, 147, 148, 151; Preville, 148, 151; Quebec City, 123, 127, 153; Quebec Province, 123, 135; Rocky Mountains, 127, 175; Royal Ottawa Golf Club, 149; Ruby Foos Chinese Restaurant, 147; Sherbrooke Street, 126, 132, 134; St Lawrence River, 123, 125, 139, 141, 148; St Matthias Church, 126, 149; Stanley Park, 176; Toronto, 136, 146, 148, 152, 175, 176; Vancouver, 147, 151, 175, 176; Vermont, 139; Westmount, 126, 132, 135, 138; **Ceylon**, 75; **China**; Shanghai, 78; **Egypt**, 60; Port Said, 77; Pyramids, 78; **Equator**, 76; **Europe**, 77, 78, 208, 209, 234; **Fiji**, 176; **France**, 41, 78, 79, 234; Marseilles, 78; Meribel, 234; Paris, 108; **Holland**, 212; **Iberian Peninsula**, 80; **Iceland**, 122; Reykjavik, 122; **India**, 208, 233; **Indian Ocean**, 74; **Ireland**, 122; **Italy**; Isle of Capri, 77; Mt Vesuvius, 77; Naples, 78; Pompeii, 77; **Mexico**, 258; **Nepal**, 208; **New Zealand**, 214; **Norway**, 234; Andennes, 234; Poland, 41; **Samoa**, 220; **Scandinavia**, 234; **Spain**, 212; Malaga, 212; **Suez Canal**, 77; **Switzerland**; Geneva, 234; **Thailand**, 183, 209, 234; Bangkok, 234; **Turkey**, 234; Gallipoli, 234; **United Kingdom**, 71, 116, 192; Australia House, 116; Ben Lomond, 98; British Titan, 236; Buckingham Palace, 93, 95, 116, 117, 120, 149; Canterbury Cathedral, 105; County Durham, 98; Covent Garden Market, 101, 106, 205; Ealing, 110; Edinburgh Castle, 99; Hampstead, 105; Hampton, 12, 105; Harley Street, 93; Isle of Skye, 100; Kenmure, 111; Lancaster House, 93, 119; London, 37, 93, 94, 95, 96, 98, 100, 101, 102, 103, 105, 107, 110, 114, 116, 117, 119, 120, 121, 125, 138, 144, 149, 203, 205, 209, 227, 234, 236; Nottingham, 119; Oldbury-on-the-Hill, 109; Pall Mall, 93; Piccadilly Circus, 93, 104; Rob Roy Pass, 98; Rock of Gibraltar, 80; Rotherhithe, 113; Scarborough, 143; Scotland, 96, 97, 98, 100, 111; Sidcup, 236; Southampton, 69, 93; St Albans, 93, 94, 96, 97, 100, 103, 110, 111, 112, 118, 119, 121, 122, 236; St Andrews Golf Links, 99; St James Palace, 93; Strand Palace Hotel, 100, 114; Stratford, 96, 97; The Savoy, 95; The Strand, 95, 104, 114, 118; Wales, 32; Westminster Abbey, 116, 117; Westminster Cathedral, 105; Windsor Castle, 105; Yorkshire, 98; **USA**, 114, 129, 234; Florida, 139; Hampshire, 139; Hawaii, 128, 176; Hollywood, 176; Las Vegas,

142; Los Angeles, 209; Manhattan Island, 145; San Francisco, 176; White Plains, 143

Transport: Airlines; Qantas, 70; Trans Australian Airlines, 70; **Ships;** SS Orcades, 175; SS Orion, 177; SS Oronsay, 74; SS Otranto, 69

Work: ANZ Bank, 46; Australian Tioxide Products, 149, 181, 187, 189, 201, 216; Bank of Australasia, 46, 59; Bank of Nova Scotia, 47, 138; Bell Telephone Company, 136; British Hawker Siddley Group, 147; Burnie High School, 203; Burra Motor Company, 9; Canadian Car and Foundry, 147, 175; Elder Smith & Co, 53; Flowercards, 229; Rodenprint, 229; Foundation Company, 125, 132, 137, 147, 149; Goldsborough Mort Stock & Station, 49; Laporte Australia, 97, 216, 235; Massey Ferguson, 175, 178, 179; National Bank, 49, 67; Parklands High School, 213; SA Brewery Co, 25, 47; United Amusement, 146, 149

Noisy birds alert
gathering storm clouds
　　　　... burst forth
quench the thirsty earth

www.ingramcontent.com/pod-product-compliance
Lightning Source LLC
Chambersburg PA
CBHW050855160426
43194CB00011B/2166